The unexpected journey,
100lbs in 100 days.

BIG SEXY FAT CAMP

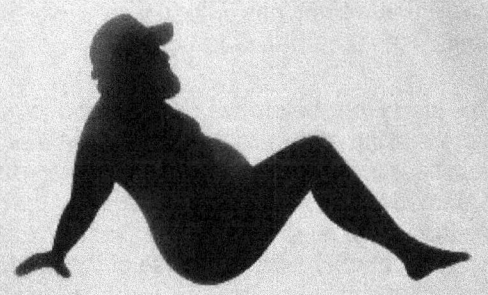

Weightloss through the eyes of a
fat guy.

Written by, Paul Frendo

Dedicated to everyone that ever stuck with me through thick and thin.
My Family, both in Michigan and Nevada.
My sisters Donna, for her inspiration and Marie for the opportunity to get healthy.
And my Brother in Law Rick for challenging me to stay on course at Fat Camp.

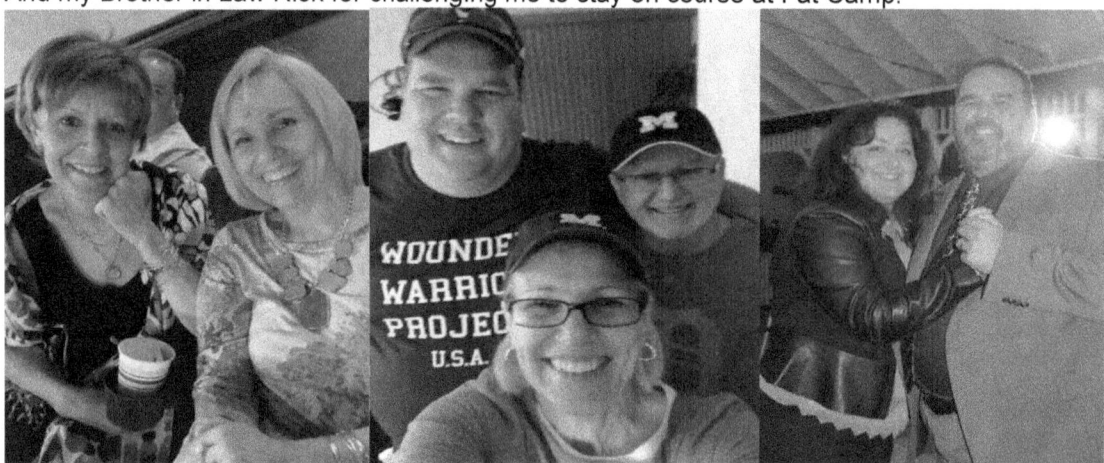

Disclaimer: First, before I offend you and you feel like closing this book, I would like to thank you and commend you on taking another chance at weight loss. I hope with every ounce of my body that this is the last time you need to start a weight loss program. Good Luck!!!

The lawyers have made me add this disclaimer before we can proceed to the meat and potatoes of this book. No animals were harmed in the making of this book, except for the ones that we eat on a regular basis. Any exercise plan should be discussed with your doctor prior to starting any exercise program. Weight loss programs are not guaranteed to work and results may vary from participant to participant. The writer of this book as well at as the publisher and everyone that has ever participated in any way shall be held harmless for any mishaps that may occur because of the following program.

This ain't coming from no profit, just an ordinary man!! In the immortal words of my favorite singer Garth, "this ain't coming from no profit, just an ordinary man." I just need a second and even a third chance to explain the reason for this book. I did not go on this journey as a fundraising mission. I went on it as a last-ditch effort to get healthy. I didn't realize how bad I was health wise until I arrived in Vegas. I guess I would have to call B.S. on myself for that statement. We drove to Vegas, the fact that I had to sit shotgun, the whole trip there, because I couldn't fit in the back seat and the fact that I couldn't walk to the bathroom when we stopped in the mountains in Utah, without assistance might have tipped me off it was bad. I never expected that the pool at the Resort Villas would be my fountain of youth. Who could have predicted that 111 days ago, I would be down over 100 lbs. and still losing? Not me!! Remember this is the guy that has been obese for over 30 years. B.S. call number two. This has been my diabolical plan since I was a kid. Hey let's play the part of a fat guy for most of your life, to the point of almost dying and get yourself to over 400 lbs. then take a trip to Vegas and lose a quarter of yourself in 100 days. I would have gotten away with it, if the meddling stroke wouldn't have happened messing up everything. Oh, ya, and then you need to write a book about the journey, because that's how you have spent your entire life as a writer. Wait, wait there's more. Make it a weight loss book since you have all these medical degrees and you are a certified trainer and a dietician. Did I nail it yet? I feel that I'm missing something, maybe Don Pardo in the background saying, "that's not all, we will throw in a set of Ginsu, steak knives just for playing along." Now I think I am done. The cherry on the top of my fat assed life. So, no, that is the unexpected part of this unexpected journey in the 50th and 51st years of my life. I didn't know until about May of 2016, that I would be spending the summer on the face of the sun with my sister Marie in Vegas. She didn't even buy the place until April of 2016. When we got there in June, it was the first time she ever stayed there, we spent the first two days unpacking and setting up her house. So, in case any of your conspiracy theorist are out there trying to crack the Davinci code on this whole sham. This book is a collection of my rants from a lifelong fat guy, that has been a product of the decades and has partaken in some very unhealthy eating practice over the years and is trying to share his pitfalls with whomever wants to listen to them. My main message from page one, is it is never too late until you take that proverbial dirt nap, to change your stars and try to get healthy. The fact that I care about my fellow fat man and woman, is irrelevant. That is my God spin on everything, I have spent pretty much my entire adult life working with kids in some aspect of my life. I should say the protection of kids. A child doesn't ask to come into this world, to the situation that they are put into. As a parent of three, it is our job to guide them to the best life we possibly can. We try to keep them healthy, happy, and safe, but unfortunately for them and for us, we forget one of the major factors in all our lives and that is nutritional factor. We don't teach them how to eat right and that is not our fault entirely, we teach them what we were taught and the cycle continues. We are also products of the generation we were brought up in. Notice I didn't say VICTIM!! I hate that word, yes unfortunately there are sick people out there that prey on the innocent or unprotected. But I am a firm believer that we can eliminate a huge percentage of victims out there if they do a better job of not putting themselves in that bad situation in the first place. Now before you look to lynch this fat guy, read what I said first and not what you think you heard. I can hear it now, "did you hear what that fat guy said?" "Rape victims deserved it." I never said anything even remotely close to that. What I did imply though is if that young lady wasn't walking by herself in an unlit bad part of town after dark, the chances of her getting assaulted would have been much lower. There is a difference, just saying. Back to my story you will find other facts, that I don't have any medical degrees, counseling degrees, dietary certificates, or professional training under my belt. I do give a lot of advice. I consider myself a self-proclaimed expert on being fat. I have over 40 years of that, so I think that qualifies me. I am a three-year survivor of a massive stroke that kept me hospitalized for nearly a month. I have been in physical therapy for almost three years, and I have been working out on and off since middle school, nearly 40 years ago, I learned to walk when I was a year old and again when I was 48. I had to relearn pretty much everything at 48. I have weighed over 400 lbs. before I decided to make the life change and take this journey at age 50 nonetheless. So, before you take everything that I just wrote and everything that I have written in this book so far and try to rip it to shreds. Let me save you the trouble and tell you to close the book, stay fat and thank you for the donation. Because, unless you were the extra three sizes in my shoes that I left in Vegas, I have no use for your negativity in my life. I have spent the last 112 days of my life trying to figure out how this 51-year-old fat stroke survivor has transformed himself from over 400 lbs. to just under 300 lbs. Basically on my own, without the use of surgery or drugs? If you can supply me with these answers, that would be helpful to me, other than that, if you would like to share my story with someone that might need to be motivated to choose life again, please do!! The other thing you will learn about me, is my overwhelming ability to jump around in my storytelling, I blame this on my non-diagnosed, A.D.D., A.D.H.D., C.R.S. and Fat Guy Syndrome. I think that covers it, for you smart, skinny people reading along so your fat guy has someone to hold his Cheetos and beer, while he flips the pages. C.R.S. stands for "can't remember shit." It is very common in fat people. Remember we can't remember when we ate last, how much we ate and when we need to eat again. But is it time to eat because I'm hungry already. Lol I do have fat fingers by the way, so sometimes my brain works faster than I can type, so I think that is why I jump around so much. Excuses, excuses, stick around I have a million of them, stories? No excuses. I feel like Willy Wonka, getting ready to open the gates to Wonka land. What's Wonka Land, said no fat person ever. That was a fat test for all the skinny people that might be peaked at this book. The gates are open, please enjoy.

This is my journey; I hope this book will inspire you to take your own journey to a healthier life. The following is a bunch of stories that document my journey through life as a fat guy. How I ended up where I started, the middle and where I ended this current journey. This book in no way is the end all be all on weight loss. I still am confused on how I could go from over 400 lbs. down to 300 lbs. in 100 days. The biggest message I would like to share with everyone is it is not too late to choose life and to decide to get healthy. If a 51-year-old 400 lb. stroke survivor with balance and vision issues can lose weight. I would challenge you to do the same. Good luck and Godspeed on your journey.

Fat Camp Tip #1, If you're just interested in how you can lose the weight fast forward to the last page of the book.

First things first.

So, first things first, who am I and what the hell do I know about health and fitness? Good questions, I consider myself a master at nothing and a connoisseur of everything. I have been in the athletic world all my life and the restaurant world for about as long. You would think with all that knowledge I never would have turned fat in the first place. turned fat, that's a funny phrase. It's like one of those social issues you see on Facebook, did you hear about Paul, he turned fat!! Hahahahahah just like that I turned fat, couldn't have been all the unhealthy food choices I made or all the time I didn't spend working off those unhealthy choices, could it? I just one day turned fat. Maybe we just decide one day to turn fat, that must be what it is. So, I am getting off the subject. I have worked with kids for a long time. I used to train baseball and softball players. In that awkward, respect kinda way some of my more seasoned smart ass players started calling me "Big Sexy" and I guess since I have pretty much been fat it stuck with me. I guess it was better than calling me fat ass, Right. As my organization grew and the more of my players adapted to calling me "Big Sexy" I guess I didn't mind that much. I also consider myself the only "Big Sexy" in West Michigan. Lol I guess the initials B.S. that you will see through the book could have a double meaning, to me they mean bull shit! But for any youngsters out there it could just mean Big Sexy says. Lol Another thing you will see throughout the book are ah ha moments. These are the moments throughout the day/week that tend to have you stopping in your tracks and leave you saying "I never thought of it that way" or "that makes sense." So, I will be adding in those occasionally also. How about now in fact. I have a section in the book about looking the part, so here is an ah ha moment for you. I was working out in the pool today and the place I work out at has several classes scheduled daily. Today being a Saturday I didn't expect the regular trainer to be there, because she already pretty much lives there Monday thru Friday. So, to my surprise when I saw a larger woman come in to instruct the water aerobics class. The first thing I was thinking is B.S.!! How do you feel qualified to teach this class? I am sure you are a real nice person and all but unless you just lost a ton of weight and are looking to be inspirational I'm not buying it. I also feel this way about genetically altered Barbie dolls that need a double cheeseburger instead of losing weight. Just saying!! Yes, you are much nicer to look at, but unless you got in that shape naturally, it's hard to take advice from someone that had the fat all sucked out. Again, just because I have walked in your shoes, maybe even bigger shoes, doesn't make me an expert, it just makes me someone that has been there done that and so far, have lived to tell about it. I am just hoping that if I can keep you from falling into some of the pitfalls that swallowed me up. This might just help you. Did you know weight loss is 80% nutrition based and 20% exercise? I have heard that more than once when I talked to a couple of trainers this week at the club. It made sense to me, because I have worked harder in my lifetime then I have worked on this last journey but have never seen this kind of result. This time I have focused just as much on the food I have shoved in the huge hole underneath my nose and just above my chin. I can honestly say that this is the reason for the success so far. Eliminating empty calories, portion control, no pop and sweets have worked wonders for me. Remember everyone is different, so you need to experiment with menu items till you find something that works for you. Every diet plan doesn't work all the time, that is another reason I hate yes, I used the hate word, DIETS!!! To truly make a difference you need to make a lifestyle change. Practice saying that, so whenever anyone asks you how you lost so much weight, you need to tell them you made a lifestyle change. It even sounds healthier!!!

It's your Body!!! The choice is yours, lose weight or don't lose weight or keep chasing that elusive miracle cure for fatness, that doesn't exist. Maybe you can wait till one is invented? Maybe you will be dead first? Stay up late and watch all the infomercials on the next great diet plan, or make a deal with your body to get healthy now. Deal with my body? What? How many times have you said to yourself, just ten more steps and we will be done? Just get me thru today and we will rest tomorrow? We have all done it. Why not make a deal with it now? I did, no I didn't talk to it but subconsciously thru my healthy choices and exercise, I said I will stop dumping shit down my throat and exercise more and make better healthy choices and start listening better too my body. You would be surprised how your body will respond when you start taking care of it. Feed it when it's hungry, rest it when it's tired give it the nutrients it needs to recover and it will do the rest. Trust me if it doesn't like what you are doing to it, then it will let you know. Piss it off too much and it will order up a dirt nap sooner than later. I reward my body at least twice a day with a trip to the hot tub. It loosens up my muscles and allows me to work out longer. I take supplements to help it heal faster, I use rubs and lotions to keep it hydrated and flexible. Whatever it needs I try to supply it. How else could an old fat stroke survivor lose 100LBS in 100 days?

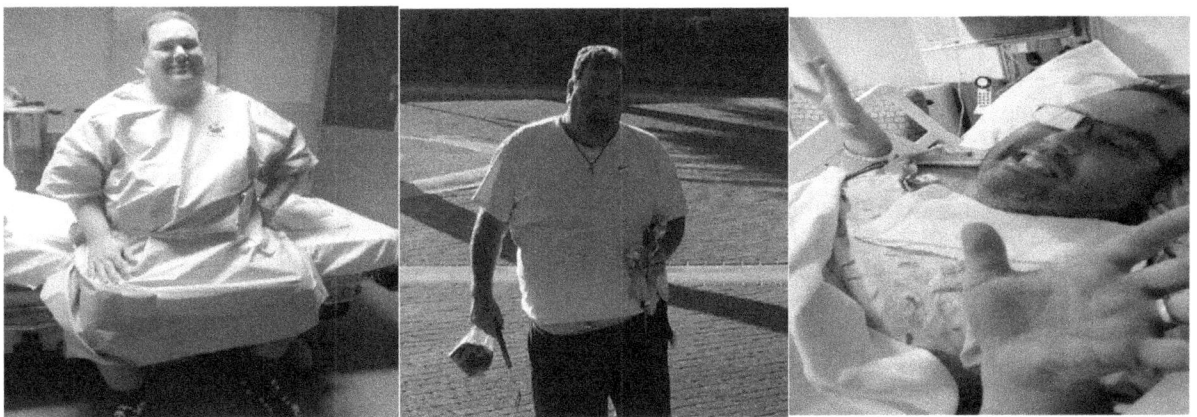

So, I'm a bit of a conspiracy theorist, when it comes to weight loss. I'm a firm believer that everyone is different and everybody doesn't process food the same way. You must choose, to fight and even kill to get healthy. No I don't mean the skinny girl again, I mean Kill cravings, calories and cheating before it kills you. You are in the fight of your life, if you don't believe that, this is not the program for you. This is not the next diet to hit the market that you can fail at. This could be the last chance you ever get to get healthy again. Make the choice to move, eat real food, drink water and see results. Getting back to that conspiracy part, who instilled our eating patterns that we are so set in our ways to break the pattern? It was probably a skinny person, because a fat person would have made the first meal of the day the biggest. Instead most people either skip the first meal or eat some fast crap to satisfy the establishment that they followed the protocol. I challenge you to step out of the norm and make your own rules. It's your body, it's your life take ownership of it. For as long as I remember breakfast was between 7am and 9am, then lunch at noon, then dinner at 6 ish. Or whenever you got home from work and the later you ate the crappier the meal was for you. Sound, about right? It is freaking 2016 why are we still following this archaic practice. It is a proven fact that people function better when the eat a nutritious meal early in the morning. They never even mention lunch, that is just a void to usually run errands and cram something down your pie hole. It is also proven that the more time you give yourself to digest the food you eat at dinner, the better it is for you. Am I lying? Yet we keep doing the same ol shit and expecting our bodies to respond to whatever we do to it. Here's a novel idea, how about going to bed a little earlier, so you can wake up a little earlier and make something more nutritious to start your day off? If you do that you probably wouldn't need to take lunch at noon. Maybe you do a healthy snack for lunch and get a quick walk in instead. Then if you are fortunate enough to be able to have a full meal early like 4pmish you give your body time to digest before you go to bed. They make a thing called a DVR if you need to watch the Tonight show that bad. Again, we are talking about your life here God forbid you don't catch the late news that is just recycled crap from the 6pm news. The longer you live in a skinny person's world the longer you will stay fat. Listen to your body and give it what it wants. Just saying!!! Don't forget also that many diet plans state that grazers lose more weight if you eat healthy snacks every four hours. I'm a firm believer of this also, you need to build a trust between you and your body. If your body feels you are going to starve it then it will turn into a hoarder until it feels it is getting enough to sustain itself between meals. You are going to ask a lot from it over your journey, reward it and keep it happy.

Conspiracy continued: If you are offended easily, again I am sorry for what you are about to read. The following is my journey to hopefully a healthy finish line in a lifelong battle to a healthy weight and body. At this point in my life TOUGH LOVE is the only way I can describe this journey. We are told a million times admitting you have a problem is the first step to solving your problem. Well I'm FAT!!! I'm not husky, full figured, big boned, plus size, large. I'm FAT!!! We live in a society of political correctness to the point of disaster. If we sugar coat it enough then maybe it will be OK, yes as a society we have evolved to accommodate fat people, we make bigger seats, bigger cloths, bigger furniture, and of course bigger portions. I guess the skinny people figured if you can't change them then accommodate them, right. Fat people have a lower life expectancy than fit people, so let's make as much money as we can off them as soon as possible, they could be dead tomorrow RIGHT!! Before you jump on my bandwagon and start blaming the fit people for us being fat, that's not where I am going with this rant. Make no mistake,

WE MADE OURSELVES FAT!!! nobody held a gun to our head and said eat fatty eat. We followed the man's guidelines and didn't listen to our bodies. We got so far out of shape and overweight that we stopped listening to what our bodies needed. I don't know about you but I ate the little devils that popped up over my shoulder, you know the red one and the white one. The red one telling you go ahead eat it won't matter and the white one telling you no stop you will regret it. So, to show that I'm an equal opportunity fat guy, I ate them both, the red one was spicy and the white one was bland in case you were wondering but nevertheless they are gone out of my life. When I chose to take this journey, it was my decision alone to do it. Yes, I had help from my family to get to where the journey began but I had to choose LIFE for any of this to be possible. Trust me if someone said to you "hey how would you like to spend the summer in Vegas with me" how hard would it be for you to say HELL YES!!! I know you would have said no, thank you, palm trees are boring the pool is probably cold and there's nothing to do there, said no one EVER!! Now add it's at a self-imposed fat camp and you're going to work your ass off literally. I see a lot of hands going down. Stay with me people, let me win you back from the fat side, everything I have done so far is low or no impact, most of it is done in the pool and you can still eat regular food. Am I getting warmer, did I peak your interest? I hope so because that is exactly what I did to lose 100lbs in 100 days.

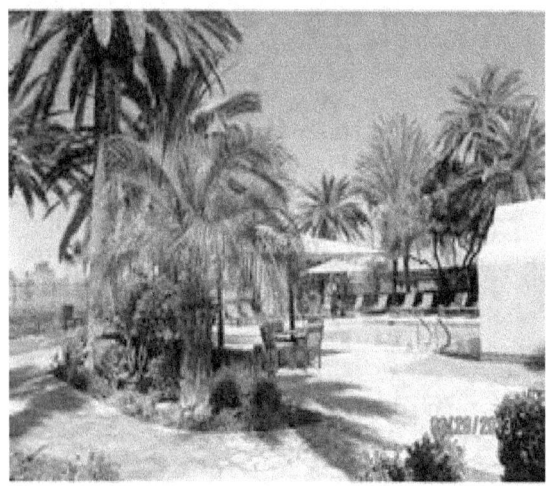 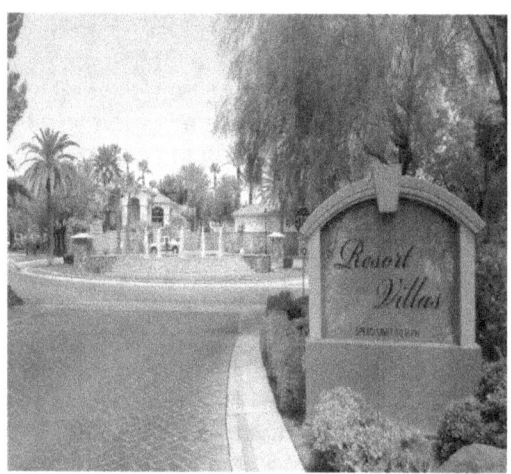

The fine print: If you are like me, you have been screwed on this little misleading tidbit once or twice. In big bold letters, they say something great, but in tiny little letters somewhere on the same document, there is the fine print basically disqualifying everything good about the bolded statement. Case in point, I'm gonna throw Yonkers under the bus. My wife and I were there last weekend for their big everything is 25% off sale. You know that magical friend and family special they run just before the holidays officially kick off. My wife thought it might be a good time to start some Christmas shopping. When low and behold, we were walking through the appliance department and we came across a Newave Air Fryer. just like the one Chef Claude bought off QVC. So, after some discussion about the pros and cons to it again, we thought it was a good price at $99.00 with the discount of 25%, heck ya $75 would make it well worth it. The wife even had an addition 10% coupon for items over $50.00 so I was feeling jolly, seeing that we were buying this gift for us, until, da, da, da!!! (eerie music) the fine print happened. We get to the register and the young lady rings it up and wtf $106.00 say what? What happened to the Everything 25% off or the additional 10%? Then the infamous words come out, Appliances are excluded from the sale and this item is already discounted, so you can't use the additional coupon either. Well, so much for my air fried chicken wings for the game Sunday or any of the other items we were thinking about purchasing that night. To say I was a little upset, is an understatement. No this is not a matter of national defense or anything like that, but this is the kind of stuff I would love the government to intervene on our behalf. Companies should not have the right to mislead their customers with false advertising and false claims, to hook them into their stores and then pull the rug out from under them, once they hook them in. You would think at age 51, I would be smarter than that, and know if it sounds too good to be true, than it probably is.

I guess I am just too trusting that someday they will just be honest with us and we will get exactly what it is they are offering us, when we decide to shop at their establishments. So, what does this have to do with weight loss, Fat Guy? Everything, I told you from the beginning most of us never look at the labels, we shop with our stomachs and pay for it with the extra weight on our bodies. I think the even worse part, is if we looked at the labels would we be able to understand them? Here is a little ditty I picked off the FDA website on labels.

Can you feel the love tonight? OK FAT PEOPLE, let's bring some love back into the conversation, I don't have a PHD in anything. I do consider myself an expert in FAT though. I have spent most of my adult life fat. When I graduated high school, I was the lowest weight of my adult life at 6'2 190 lbs. It didn't take long to climb into the 200's by my early 20's. My weight increased gradually as my activity level dropped. I spent most of my 20's in the restaurant world so long hours and horrible eating habits. I started college at age 30 and spent the early part of my 30's as a college student. Upon graduation with a business administration degree I entered the banking world. Again, long hours, combined with poor eating habits and low activity was the perfect storm when it came to weight gain, it was then that entered into the 300's. When I hit the 300's the first time, I felt a call of urgency to lose weight. I will bore you with more of how that story played out later in the book. For now, let's get back to the love. It's time to interject a B.S. Call here, ALL!! Fat people sit around all day and eat ice cream and surf Facebook. Did I nail it? That's what we all do right. Problem solved stop eating ice cream log off Facebook and get a job, follow those three tips and you will be cured of your fatness. Let me break it down for any of you skinny people looking for a way to drop from a size 4 to a 0. Fat people started out just like you but for most of us something happened in our life that helped make us like this. Maybe it's genetics, low metabolism, depression, an injury and so on and so on and so on!!!! let's see by a show of hand who was born and the first words out of your mouth was I want to be fat. Or better yet when people asked you what you wanted to be when you grew up, you said "FAT" said no fat person EVER. So then why are so many of us? Did you not get the memo you have to be cool to be fat!!!! Ahhhhhhhhhh wrong answer!!! nobody asks to be fat, it's something that happened.

Rule number 3 at fat camp: YOU CAN'T CHANGE THE PAST BUT YOU CAN CHANGE YOUR FUTURE. I use the word journey a lot in this book because life's a journey, it is filled with ups and downs, good and bad things. The journey is not over till you reach a destination. In life, the end of the destination is death, would you like to help control the journey or have someone else control when you check out?

Tip # 1 @ Fat Camp: That brings me to my first lesson at fat camp. No one can do this for you!! This has to be all you. Yes, they can support you, they can encourage you but ultimately it is up to you. Most of my journey is by myself, I started out being in the pool 15 mins, to an hour, then went three to four hours a day and by the end of my time in Vegas, I was up to eight to ten hours a day at a time usually without anyone else within miles of me it seemed. For me this is the perfect workout. I can work at my pace; I don't have to work around anyone and most of all I don't have to stop what I'm doing to make small talk. Don't get me wrong human interaction isn't a bad thing, but when you are on a mission the last thing you need is a distraction. I am not a big fan of bringing my phone with me too the pool. First of all because a week into my journey I forgot it was in my pocket and it did my work out with me, I was without a phone for three weeks waiting for a replacement. The second reason is because it never fails, you get deep into a workout and your phone will go off and most of the time it is a useless call. Third and the only reason I ever take my phone is because I am fat and I have health issues, I have two strikes against me God forbid I had an issue and had to call 911 I would never make it if I didn't have my phone. So, for that reason I usually bring it, I don't ever answer it unless it rings repeatedly then it better be an emergency on the other end of the line. Remember this is your time for your health... This is your time for you. Shut down your mind, forget your to do list, stop thinking of all the bull shit that happened at work that day and focus on what a healthy life would feel like. I hear a huge B.S coming. It's easy for you to say, you don't have my life to deal with and I say with a resounding hell to the yes!!! I have my own demons to contend with then to deal with yours too. Ever hear the saying don't sweat the small stuff? Focus on the stuff that you can change stop worrying about the stuff you can't? Sound familiar. Again, I still hear the B.S. chants coming from the peanut gallery. I'm telling you until you exercise the demons out of your life they are going to hold you back from your goal of getting healthy. I guess you are wondering how I achieved this, I haven't completely. It is a work in progress, it is mind over matter. I don't mind because it doesn't matter.

Again, I only worry about what I can change, focus on figuring out a solution and taking care of the problem. There are things out there like death and taxes that we know will be with us forever, why worry about them they are always going to be out there lurking. I don't worry, I can only pay the things I have money for and if I am working to get healthy I am pissing off the grim reaper too. So how come it is, we keep putting things off until later? Later today, later this week, later this year, Ok maybe even next year. We do that a lot with health issues. You have a bad back, or shoulder or knee. We know it needs to be fixed, but we would rather live in pain then to take the time out of our busy schedules to get the problem fixed. We do the same thing with our weight. I will watch what I eat next time. Or I will start a diet next week. The longer we put it off, the more weight we gain until we end up saying screw it, I need to lose so much weight, I will never be able to do it so why try? Been there done that. So, since we are keeping it real, I need to fess up. On the same note the laser focus pertains to the beginning of your journey. Don't forget I used to be alone in the pool sometimes for up to 10 hours. Being alone for that amount of time gives you plenty of times to hash things through your brain and sort some things out. Again, if you are limited on time to work out, please try to clear your head and listen to your body. Music works well to help with that as well as meditation. I know nothing about meditation but I have been told by some skinny people that it works for them. lol

The Beginning: First things first, remember I am not a doctor or a dietitian or a trainer. I do not have any initials behind my name indicating that I know anything more than any other overweight smart ass, product of the sixties does. The following stories are a description of my life and how I got to be in the place and state that I currently reside on this planet. This book is not designed to change your life or even give you anymore hope then you had before you opened it to read it. My only message to you is that it's never too late until you are dead to make a change for the better. Also, if you are skinny why the hell are you wasting your time reading this book, beware fat people hate skinny people that think they are fat and are always on diets. Rule number one in this book is if you see a skinny person reading this book EAT THEM!!! If the police, ask you why you ate them tell them because they were skinny not because I told you to eat them. Now that we got that out of the way we can begin. Once upon a time there lived a little fat kid named Paulie, it may not be politically correct to use the word fat but since it is me I felt OK saying it. If that word offends you, then you might want to stop reading this book. We have watered down the truth so much as to not offend anyone by labeling them with new terms that are so damn confusing we don't know what we are. I guess I could call myself nutritionally deficient and intolerant or eliminating calories if that works for you but for the sake of argument I'm fat. I have been fat pretty much all my life, even as a child I was husky. Gotta love that term too Husky that too is a term used to not offend a child that is fat. We as adults are responsible for our children. Buying them bigger cloths is no excuse for eating right in the first place. I'm getting off topic I tend to do that sorry I'm not Dr. Phil. So, going thru life as a fat kid is not a walk in the park. I guess I should clarify the term "fat kid" I wasn't obese by today's standards but growing up I had love handles and man boobs, so I guess that qualifies me as a "fat kid" as well as I loved cake and dessert in general and unless we were bad that day we always ended dinner time with dessert. I guess this would be a good spot to interject a B.S. Call. How many of you have heard this before? "You have to finish everything on your plate" before you are done. If you didn't you had to hear about all the starving kids in Ethiopia!!! So, since we are a society that feels better about pointing fingers at people that made us this way, I guess I will point my finger at my parents. I'm fat because my mother made good food that I loved to eat and it's my dad's fault because he would beat our ass if we wasted any of it. Does any of the sound familiar? We carried this on for generations and probably used it on our kids as well. Here is tip number one. Put down your fork when you are full. If at all possible throw the unused portion away, so to not be tempted to eat it later in the same day. No, I'm not saying waste tons of food, learn to take only what your gonna eat at that meal. You can plan on leftovers for the next day but that should be food that has not been on your plate, guilting you to eat me because you know you want too!! There is a difference. Portion control is key. Here is another helpful tip I learned from my Nephew and his Fiancé, when they go out to dinner they never bring leftovers home. They eat all they want while they're at the restaurant and leave the remains there. This eliminates the late-night cravings to eat again something probably high in calories. Here's a fat test for you. How many of you love pizza, so the average person would have trouble eating a small pizza by themselves so instead of a small we order an extra-large so we can take the leftover pizza home for breakfast right, how many times have you not had pizza left for breakfast because you had a midnight snack? Healthy, right? Not. OK so now that we have established that it's our parents fault for us being fat, what do we do? Most of us do nothing right, because who wants to prosecute your parents am I right? We go thru life flying by the seat of our pants ignoring what our doctors say and what our bodies are telling us until we hit that proverbial wall right. Did you know weight loss products are a multibillion with a B business? It blows my mind that we can walk on the moon, have cars that drive them self, communicate with people instantly around the world but we don't have a pill that can keep us at the ridiculous weight to height formula the doctor's office has so graciously set for us. I'm a product of the 60's I believed in the Jetson's that by the 2000's we would have things in place for weight maintenance and that was my plan B. So now I have another thing to blame my fatness on cartoons. You seeing a trend here yet? There is always someone or something we can blame our weight problem on. If you think about it WEIGHT PROBLEM could be an oxymoron for most of us, because I don't know about you I have no problem gaining weight. I also can think of tons of excuses why I can't succeed losing weight so why even start trying right? This brings me to the reason I started my self-imposed fat camp. As I mentioned earlier most people need a life changing event to happen for them to seriously make a change for the good. Here I am going thru life as a fat guy doing everything I can to support my family. I am 48 years old have a wife and three great kids, I own two businesses, work at another plus substitute teach a couple of days a week in my free time right. It is right after Christmas break the kids go back to school and I get a head cold from one of the germ magnets that I was substitute teaching. I had had ringing in my left ear for years. My doctor and I had written it off as Tinnitus for years but the cold pretty much made me deaf in my right ear as well. My new doctor wanted me to investigate it further and scheduled me with an ENT and an MRI later they discovered that I had an acoustic neuroma at the base of my brain stem. On the bright side if you're gonna get a brain tumor this is the one you would want, it was be-nine so that was a plus also. This was diagnosed in March of 2013, I got a couple of surgical options and settled on a surgery date of December 3. 2013. For all accounts the surgery was going to last 6-8 hours I would be in recovery for 2 hours then moved to my room where I would stay in the hospital for five days then be released to home on restricted duty for up to 30 days so that is what I prepared for. I guess that was the normal person's picture but the fat guy scenario changed dramatically. The surgery took 11 ½ hours from the operating room to ICU I went into a hypertensive crisis (stroke) I was in ICU for five days in the hospital for an additional three days then shipped to a rehabilitation hospital for almost a month, where I had eight hours of physical therapy, occupational therapy and speech therapy a day. I went into the rehab hospital in a wheelchair and came out with a walker. I was basically taken back to square one. I had to relearn pretty much everything, yes, my brain knew how to do everything but my body didn't know how to perform it.

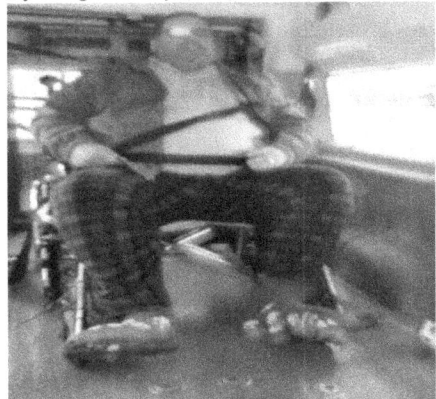 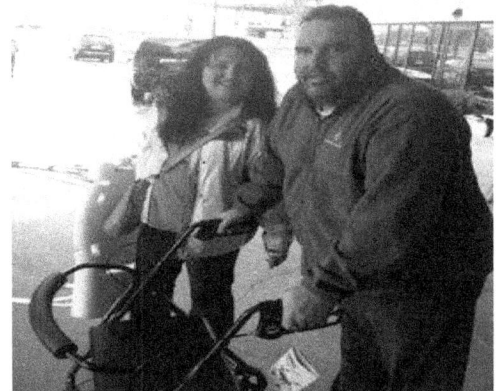

So, OK fast forward to February 2014 in Michigan I am still doing therapy three times a week, we have about two feet of snow on the ground. My weight is about 375 by this time. I am taking seven pills a day of assorted medication. What would you do? I went thru the stages of grief on a daily basis. It would have been so easy to just sit on that couch and wait to die then to go thru everything that I have gone thru the past three years. Let me remind you why I didn't choose to end it then. I had a wife that was by my side that whole ugly journey the support of my family, friends, and players to think of. Players you say? I'm sorry I failed to mention that one of the business's I owned was a sports training facility of which I trained several hundred ball players that played baseball and softball on my travel teams. So yes, I had an obligation to them also, which made it pretty much impossible to give up.

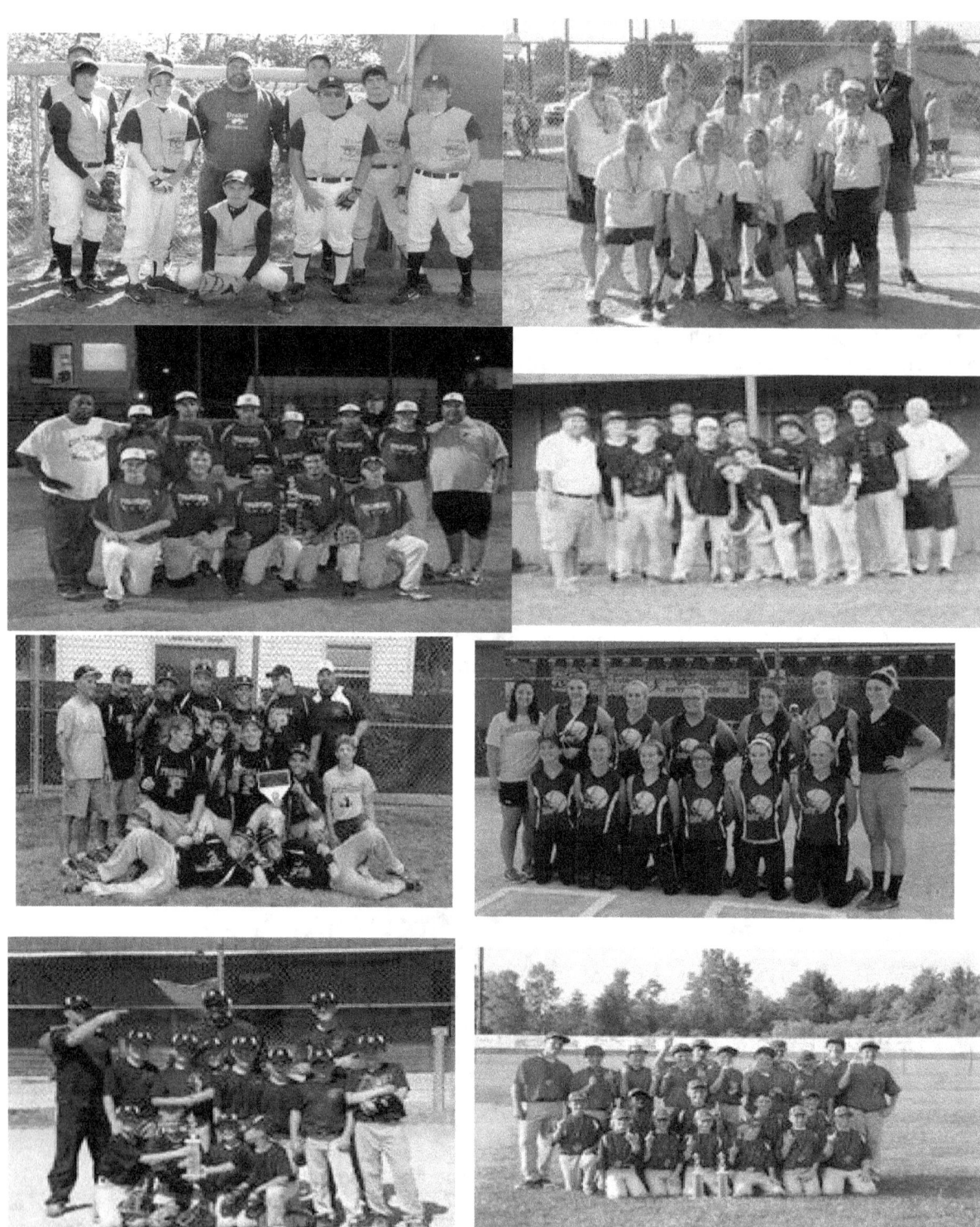

I learned at a young age that life is full of choices and every choice you make there is something attached to that choice you make; it may be good or it may be bad based on the choice you make. Here is one motto that I lived by after all I had been thru. "Life isn't worth living unless you are living your life". In the simplest of terms, if you're not truly experiencing the life you are living and just going thru the motions you are not truly living your life. There are more states that are against euthanasia then support it. So, choose to live, but live on your terms, as a stroke survivor I have chosen to live life to the fullest. No I can't do everything I might have been able to do if I hadn't had the stroke but here is my next tip. Stop trying to change the things you have no control over, take control over the things you can change.

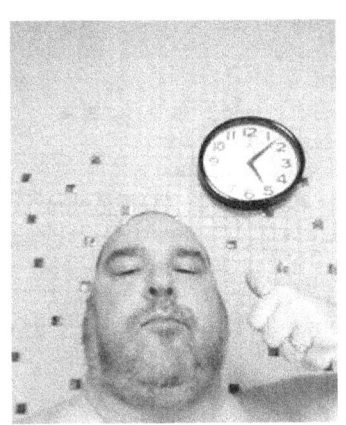

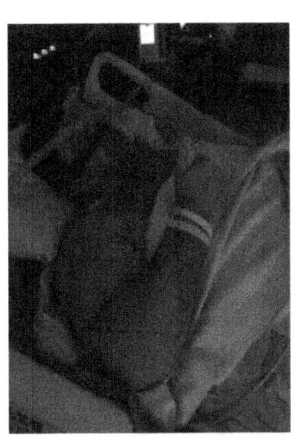

The Big Sexy 5K Challenge

Swimming 5K to help support Mary Free Bed

Thursday December 4th
With the support of The Tamarac Rehabilitation Center

Mary Free Bed

Please make donations directly to
Mary Free Bed.
The donations are tax deductible.

OK let's get back on my journey, so here I am now I am 49, still doing physical therapy three times a week. The facility that I go to therapy at is also a fitness center with a pool. So, I got a membership for the pool only. My doctor wasn't sure it was a good idea if the fat guy sweat too much yet. So, for about a year I swam two to four hours a day in that pool. I even swam 500 laps as a fundraiser for the rehabilitation hospital that I spent a month at. The work I put in at the pool made me stronger and helped me get strong enough to get rid of the walker. So now I was pretty independent and making progress but it seemed that the longer I swam it didn't equate into weight loss. It was very discouraging. On a positive note though I loved the water, being in the weightless environment just after the stroke made me feel normal again. It wasn't until I would get to the second step of the pool that gravity would kick in and the struggle to deal with land travel would begin again. The other advantage of the pool was when I lost my balance the water was a lot more forgiving than the floor was. So here I am with thousands of laps accomplished in the pool but not much to show for it on the scale, I guess this is where I need to fess up about my mental status. Remember my little rant about choices, I had pretty much come to the conclusion that my time on this planet was running low, so I decided if I was going to die anyway, I was going to die happy and not deprive myself of my guilty pleasures, cookies, ice cream, steak & potatoes. So, I didn't and pretty much all the work I was doing in the pool paid for my guilty pleasures. This brings me to spring of 2016, here I am pretty much as normal as I'm gonna be health wise, my life is getting busy. I still have time for physical therapy but not so much for the pool. So, I stop swimming. I figure I'm so busy with life that this should cover for my guilty pleasures, right? NOT! my weight climbs to an all-time high of over 400. Now combine that with all the medications I am still taking and it's a recipe for disaster. This is where a little

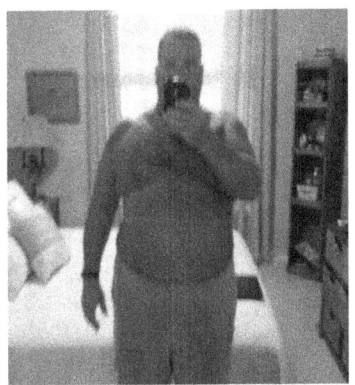

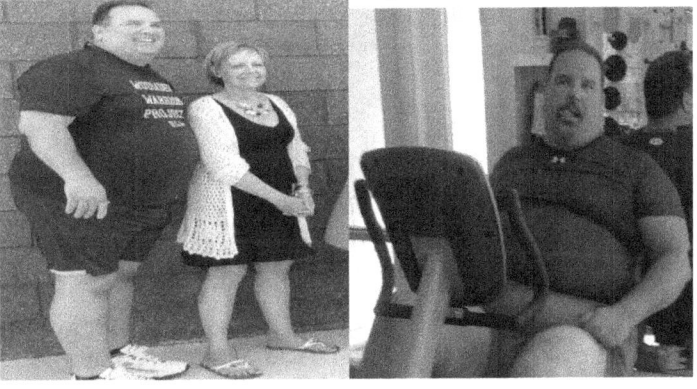

divine intervention comes in. I am the ninth child of a family of 10, eight of my siblings have struggled with their weight at some point in their life. The sister that has lived the healthiest life out of all of us has had three bouts with cancer, go figure!!! Her determination to continue to fight that awful disease has inspired me to continue to live my life. So being supportive in her fight I connected more with another one of my sisters that had recently purchased a home in Henderson Nevada and she invited me to spend the summer with her on the face of the sun as they call it. Being a disabled fat guy, it wasn't too hard to clear my schedule. That takes me to where this journey began. We drove from Michigan to Nevada; it took three days to complete the trip. We left on June 19th and arrived June 22nd. June 23rd began my first day of my self-imposed fat camp. So, as I stated earlier I have no formal training in the healthcare industry but I have been an athlete all my live as well as a coach and trainer so I do know my way around the gym. For me I don't believe in most of the diet plans out there that are based on replacing actual food. Hence protein shakes, juice cleansing, power bars, things like that. Yes, they are a great way to kick start a true health plan but if you don't have time to establish a healthy dietary meal plan that your body can survive on. The odds are so stacked against your success; you waste your time and money on it. My self-imposed fat camp is just a name that you can joke about with your friends but to you, for me it's a mission. I was asked today, what I was doing to lose weight since they noticed me always in the pool and slimming down he asked me the standard skeptical questions most cynical people such as myself would ask when someone says the words, diet, program, or lifestyle change. How many calories do you get? Did you eliminate carbs? No sugar, right? How much is that gonna cost me? My answer to him was no,no,no and whatever you want to spend and you know what he said, Bull Shit!!! right. As of today, August, 8th 2016 at 11am Pacific time I have lost 50.4 LBS in 46 days without doing any dieting. I have stop drinking soda, and eating sweets but I have had my share of Corona with lime, steak, burgers, chicken, ribs, eggplant parmigiana, and even nachos. Here it comes I feel it BULL SHIT!!! Honest to God!!! I have focused on portion control, stopped doing seconds and have chosen healthy snacks. I love watermelon and cantaloupe. I do a fruit smoothie every morning following my morning workout that consists of frozen strawberries, banana, almond milk and two scoops of whey protein to help my muscles recoup faster. But that's it, my typical day, I wake up about six am, make a peanut and jelly sandwich, drink a bottle of water go do my morning workout, come back home drink a smoothie go outside do my land walk, come back in around noon, drink another bottle of water maybe have some fruit if I'm even hungry, then about 5 pm eat a good meal. Last night I had a pork chop, sweet potato and salad, water to drink and a bowl of watermelon while I watched the Olympics. Did I count the calories? No, was it diet food? No could I eat more if I wanted to? Yes, but I'm on a mission and when you are seeing results you don't mind being focused. So, what's the catch you must be asking yourself? Right, I haven't found one yet. I am burning more calories than I am taking in. that is what I am attributing it to. I try my best to keep active, other than stopping to sync my watch and write this book, I am laser focused on burning calories. I guess maybe I do have an advantage because I am in a resort setting with the palm trees by the pool, but it is also 108 degrees pretty much all the time and the fact I have not seen my wife and kids for 50 days. Life is all aces. Lol I use the sacrifices my family and friends have made for me to come have my self-imposed fat camp as fuel to do my best at losing weight. No one said your fat you need to go do this. I chose life, it was my decision. Something you have to remember is I'm not a stranger to working out in the pool. I did it for almost three years at my local pool so I did have a routine in place when I restarted in the pool out here. No I didn't weight 400 lbs. when I was working out back in Michigan and no I didn't go 100%-gung ho when I got here either, I did a little more everyday till I hit a full week, then as my challenges increased on my Garmin I ramped up my workout regimen. The thing about working out in the pool is yes you get fatigued but I have yet to get sore from working out in the pool. Also, you have to listen to your body, if it tells you that you are tired SLEEP!! I have taken several naps in the afternoon because I am not used to taking 30,000 plus steps in a day. I have also slept in a couple days when my body wanted to sleep. It doesn't mean I didn't do my work out that day it just meant I got a later start doing the workout. There is a big difference in the two. I think the biggest tip I can give you there is, you can always do more today but you can't make up for what you didn't do yesterday. Your body also resets itself when you sleep at night, yes, you can burn extra calories today that will help burn more of what you eat today, but in my experience my body at least doesn't let me go make up for my sins in the past. Don't forget you are in a partnership with your body, you can't ask it to do more than it is willing to do. The same holds true when you lie to it, for example you might be on the treadmill and you tell yourself you're going to do three miles today, you keep telling yourself the whole time how much more you need to do to get to three miles. Then you get to three miles and decide let's do four miles instead, you have changed the game plan, yes, your body is going to do what you ask it to do, but remember that trust issue I mentioned earlier, if you go to the well too much and keep lying to yourself karma is a bitch. Why do you think people have heart attacks and strokes, because we push our bodies too hard? So be careful what you ask for that's just a tidbit of advice.

How did I get here? So how did I get here? That's a good question, how do any of us get here. Poor diet, no exercise, bad eating habits, times I ate, stress eating, physical or mental issues there are tons of ways how we got here but very few ways to get back to a healthy you. I have no initials behind my name that would make me an expert in this field. All I have is 50 years of eating and spending a majority of my life trying to shed the pounds I have gained by eating my way too here. There are many great diets, plans and programs out there you can try that may or may not work for you. In my experience, they all pretty much have pros and cons to all of them. If you are not committed 100% to getting the results you want then you will fail pretty much 100% of the time, sure in the beginning you see a result because you try your hardest in the beginning. Most of us have that same attitude "I wasted my money on this product and I want to see a result". So, we do it for a week or two then we are on to the next sensation to hit the market or we just fall back into our same ol same ol and gain double the weight we just lost. I have found that it takes a life changing event for most of us to take getting healthy a priority in our life. The sad truth to that statement is some of us don't get that second chance, many of us don't make it thru the heart attack or stroke the first time, we usually react to this life

changing event from a close family member or friend and say, I don't want the same thing to happen to me. Unfortunately, most of the time it is too late for us because by then the odds are stacked so far against us we are too set in our ways to make the changes we need to make the changes that will make the differences we need to succeed. If I had a nickel for every time I have tried a new diet or exercise plan, I would have a lot of nickels. Until this last attempt to get healthy the only thing that has ever helped me lose a major quantity of weight is DRUGS!!. Now before you all get your phones out and start looking to score some street meds. I need to clarify that statement. Back in my late 30's I was at the end of my weight rope. I was the heaviest I had ever been to that point in my life, right at about 300 lbs. I was having other physical issues also, high blood pressure, migraines, swelling in my legs and feet. Always tired, sleep apnea. I went to my family doctor at the time and we discussed my situation. He was very knowledgeable about the current prescription drugs on the market as well as the side effects both good and bad. At that point I was willing to try anything to lose weight. I must add that bariatrics was in its early stages and really not an option for me at that time. My doctor prescribed me Toprol and Bontril which were both migraine medication at the time but taken together in the early stages were very effective as appetite suppressants. For example: I started taking the medication on Thursday, by the following week it was in full effect. That following Saturday my wife and I were shopping and I had to stop her because I was having an issue, my teeth felt huge when I touched them with my tongue, I was weak and sweaty I wasn't sure what was happening. She asked me when was the last time I ate anything and I asked her what day it was. She informed me it was Saturday and I responded Tuesday. Needless to say, we quickly got some protein in me. I continued that medication protocol with additional exercise and a diet plan in place I dropped nearly 100 lbs. in three months. Needless to say, I don't remember much from those three months. Other than the weight loss the other big positive was at the end of the three month my doctor ordered my second colonoscopy to make sure everything internally was OK. For those of you that have never had the pleasure of a camera on snake devise blown up your butt that's not the best part of the whole procedure. 24 hours before your photo op, you must drink this lovely concoction called Go-lightly!! Trust me if it works for you lightly is not how it comes out of you. Getting back to the other positive to the medication I was taking was the ability to control how long I could go without eating. So, when the nurse informed me that I needed to fast for 24 hours prior to the procedure and drink this lovely product, being the smart ass that I am I replied how about I skip food for 48 hours and we call it good. Being unamused the nurse did feel that this was adequate and we went with it. Luckily for me everything was good and besides my blood pressure being a little low we were all good with the results of that test.The other significant finding I experienced thru this drug induced coma diet was the major effect carbohydrates played on my body. As the pills took their effect on my regular diet, I realized that I still had a hunger and a need for food. My issue was that as soon as I prepared the food and all the smells hit me I was nauseated after about two bites of whatever I made I couldn't eat any more, hence the continuing weight loss. I guess I should have mentioned this earlier in the book but I consider myself a barfophobic. Up until my recent health issues I could recite pretty much to the date and time I had thrown up in my lifetime, that I was old enough to remember. No I don't remember spitting up when I was being bottle fed when I was a child but I am sure if I could have I would have added them to the list. So, let's just say for the sake of argument I HATE TO THROW UP!!!!! So, this also made the drug induced diet effective on me. Because whenever I felt nauseated I would stop eating immediately. That brings me to my next discovery about my body. My body doesn't process carbs very well. I love bread, pasta and pretty much any baked goods. While on my drug diet the smell of any baked products made me want to hurl. Case in point my banking center that I worked at was in a shopping center. One of our clients, without naming names, their name sounds like tub-play bake their breads daily. It took everything I had to deliver their receipts back to them at any time of the day, without getting sick. Even more disturbing is the fact that I was on these drugs during Christmas time and I can honestly say that I DID NOT!! eat one Christmas cookie that year. I started this regiment in late November and stopped taking them in early February. The results were a resounding success I lost nearly 100lbs but I also lost about four months I can hardly remember. The other resounding negative was that I never learned any good eating habits over that time frame either so the weight came right back from which it had left me. Like I mentioned earlier, there are many great diet plans on the market. What I have found in my 30 plus years of dieting though is they are so expensive or restricting that I usually got pissed off and went back to my old ways. If you are like me let's just say "cynical" that was the nicest word I could come up with on the spot. I HATE the word DIET. Any word that derives from the word DIE rubs me the wrong way. It's kind of like a threat, even though left unattended we could die from our unhealthy lifestyle. But aren't we all superhuman and we do what we want? Pretty much!!! but we need to put on our big kid panties and rationalize with our demons. Fat camp question time, how many of us like to be told what to do? By show of hands, fingers don't count for this portion of the test. EXACTLY so why do we do it anyway? Just because it's been done this way forever doesn't mean that we can't be rebels and do it our own way. Who made them the boss of us and told us I have to eat breakfast first before 9am then lunch at noon and dinner at 6pm and of course my biggest favorite is since we are adults we should go to bed after the 11pm news or better yet after the tonight show. Here's a news flash for you people F'em. Again, they don't own me. I will do what I want when I want because I'm a grown ass person!!!! Everyone has their own demons to fight, everybody is different, maybe you're a square peg that just doesn't fit into that round hole, does that make you any less than the round person next to you? I mentioned this earlier but like me I probably wasn't listening except for the skinny girl that did not heed my warning and is risking her life to get thru this entire book without getting eaten by a fat person. When did we stop listening to our bodies? Probably around middle school, by then we knew everything pretty much and don't need any more information out there clouding our decision-making process because if you are anything like me in elementary we were still controlled by the man, sorry I mean mom, if you were fortunate enough to have a mother at home whose main duty was to pack our lunch for the day you know what I'm talking about. Sometimes we were excited for lunch cause maybe you had something good the night before and you might get a little more something something today instead of a smashed pb&j and some crushed chips. We did get to make a choice though this prepared us for the tough decisions we had to make in middle school White or Chocolate and for the rich schools Strawberry was an option. As one of the fat kids in elementary I ran the first ever that I know black market barter system for upgrading your lunchtime enjoyment. By about the fifth grade we knew the tendencies of the mother packed lunches for most of the kids in the school. For the right price, I could upgrade your boring pb&j lunch to cold pizza a candy bar and a soda. To a kid in elementary a lunch like that scored you bonus street cred, trust me on that one. Sorry for the trip down memory lane, let me get back to the root of most of our problem. Middle school lunch. For most of us this was our first opportunity to make our healthy food choices and if they gave a grade for lunch most of us would have failed. Holy crap for a fat kid this was like JACKPOT, pizza, cheeseburgers, cookies, cake, soda if I had money in my lunch account I was golden. Remember I was a product of the sixties; we didn't have guys like Jamie Oliver running around telling us how toxic the food we were consuming was affecting our future health of our body if the lunch ladies scooped enough crap on our plate to keep us happy everything is fine with us. I don't think we even need to discuss high school add open campus lunches and fast food places.... Enough said. So, let's move on shall we do after graduation and our first jobs. If it can go in a microwave we were golden. We didn't care what it tastes like if it was fast and cheap. Hence the invention or Ramen noodles. Is it just me or shouldn't there be a huge red flag up when it cost that company more for the Styrofoam cup it comes in then the product we consume out of it? Just saying. Moving on, some of us were lucky enough to find a mate and thank God for wedding showers because for some of us this was the first time since living at home that we used pots and pans and real dishes. We didn't know how to cook much but we were good fakers. We all pretty much had our go to dish when it was our turn to cook. Mine was pasta. I could open a jar of sauce with the best of them and if the noodles weren't too crunchy dinner was a success if you had a dishwasher, if not it pretty much sucked doing dishes too. Sure, over time we learned more dishes to cook and evolved into master chefs, right? OK maybe not but as we got older more restaurant chains opened so we had a plethora of healthy choices at the tip of our tongues. Right? This phase just seemed to never end and helped contribute to our growing health issues. That must be it, the restaurant chains are to blame for me being fat, right? If they didn't offer the super-size, I just would have ordered a normal size said no fat person ever!!! We have all seen the news where someone always tries to sue a chain restaurant because they made them fat!!!! News flash we made us FAT!!! there isn't a magic potion out there that gives us the munchies or is there? You know that restaurant chain that sounds like Chaco Smell has invented a fourth meal for our convenience. This brings me to my next B.S. Call; this might be a little off topic but I don't care this is my life story. Here are my messed-up hypotheses on Chaco Smells menu choices. I think a group of fat stoners meet in the back room of one of their restaurants wasted out of their minds and slap a couple of their regular menu items together slather it with nacho cheese and call it some crazy combination of names and act like they came up with the cure for hunger. Is it just me or can I get an Amen!! Sure, this new product is going to appeal to a good portion of their customer base as marijuana becomes more legalized in more states, I guess the jury is still out on that one. So back to me, I must be honest with you the part where I cooked with jar sauce was a lie. I couldn't live with myself if I didn't come clean on that one but pretty much everything else is spot on. I was raised in the restaurant business, I spent about 20 of my years owning or managing someone else's restaurant. I pretty much managed every fast food chain available at least the big ones. My favorite customer was the petite plus size person that would come thru the drive thru, I guess they must have gotten all their work in at the gym and couldn't make the long trek from the parking lot to the front counter and would order a double Whopper, large fry, and a large diet soda. Cause I guess all the sodium in the diet soda would counteract the calories consumed from the sandwich and fry's. See I understood their logic because I too was a petite plus sized food service employee. For the most part the initial food used to create your value meal started out as a viable food item minus all the preservatives, additives and cooking procedure used from commissary to your tray. When the food left the premises, all bets were off it becomes your property to do with it what you desire. If you choose to leave it in your car for a couple of hours while you run errands that is on you. Again, ownership of the problem is key here. In my 51 years on this planet I have never heard of a person being kidnapped at gunpoint and forced to drive a person to a fast food restaurant and order them a value meal super-sized and stay with their captors while they consumed it. I might be wrong but I'm pretty sure that CNN would have broken in during me Fresh Prince marathon to report this breaking crises. So now my secret is out I have over 20 years of cooking experience under my fat belt. How could I have let food do this to me? Why didn't I just cook healthy food and only consume the proper portions of this healthy food? Why do any of us let this happen? Life!!!! pretty much in a nutshell from the hours that we keep, running the kids to all their events, lack of meal planning, the convenience of take out. It could be any or all the above combined with a million other reasons. Fat people don't need much of an excuse not to eat healthy. We just need food. Now for my next B.S. Call. Fat people must sit around all day watching TV and eating bon bon's. For a majority of my life I worked like a Hebrew Slave. Working seven days a week 10 to 12 hours a day. I could run circles around most skinny people and I was carrying most of them skinny people on my back literally. That is why I suggested in the opening paragraph that we eat all the skinny people of the world cause the makeup many of the fat jokes we endure. Me not being educated in the medical field leaves me unqualified to make an educated and accurate dissertation on this matter but here I go anyway. I have said it over and over so far, everybody is different. You need to listen to your body. Stop trying to make it what it is not and what it may never be. I feel confident in this next statement. The best diet plan known to mankind will not have the same result on every person trying it!!! If it was that simple everyone would be built the same. Everyone would have blond hair and blue eyes, have an athletic build and be gorgeous. This is never going to happen because we all have a different DNA make up, we were formed by two different people then the people you are not related too, so why do we try to solve everyone's weight issues with the same fixes? So, are you ready for no more B.S and hear how I lost 100 lbs. in 100 days? I feel like Howie on Deal or no Deal, I will tell you right after this message.... Dick move right. I'm sorry

Here We Go!!!

Here's what I did!!! I told you at the beginning of the book that this was not a new miracle weight loss program or a fix all for everyone. Fat people as a bonus I did offer up skinny people as a snack while you read on. This program was designed with stroke survivors in mind. Again, everyone is different and every need is different. Let's see who was paying attention and who just skipped to this page too see my big fat secret. Here it is

CHOOSE to LIVE!!!

Wow that was simple, choose to live, why didn't you think of that? For another simple reason, Life Happens!!

Life Happens, What the hell does that mean fat guy? You know those times when unexpected things pop up out of nowhere and hit you straight between the eyes. That's life. You can prepare all you want, or be as unprepared as much as you want. Then bam! Like a lightning bolt, life happens. For example, you take care of your car, right? Oil changes, brakes, tune ups regular, then bam! You break down on the way to work in the rain, most of the time. You think WTF, or is that just me. You think, I just had this p.o.s. in the shop for a tune up. That's Piece of Shit, for those skinny Cheeto bag holding, beer holding, so the fat guy can flip the page people that may still be lurking out there. lol You get it towed into the shop. The mechanic says," Looks like you have a mouse problem." Again, WTF, he goes on to say "the little bastards crawled up under the hood and decided to feast on your wiring." Isn't that special, is it something you planned on? NO, is it something you could have prevented, maybe but probably not. Is it something you were prepared to pay for, hell to the no!! Life happens. Case number two, you and the wife getting frisky, things go a little farther than expected, should we stop and find protection? Hell, no, we are married and nine months later you're a real family now. Ready or not. Life really happened now. Were you ready for the responsibility of another life to take care of? Hard to say, but you will love that child unconditionally, right? Because life happened. There are so many reasons why we put on weight and many of them can be blamed on Life. we can't stop living because we are worried about life happening, but we can do a better job living healthier in our life. Remember life is a choice and a gift. Choose wisely, live wisely and hopefully live longer. Just saying To be successful in anything you do you have to be committed to be successful. Being and getting healthy is a choice that require total focus and total commitment and when I was put in a get healthy or die decision I chose to live and to live on my terms. You must be prepared to think outside the box and listen to your body. Not only do you have to listen, you need to follow what it is saying. Before I started my self-imposed fat camp my body was telling me I wouldn't make it too New Years. No I wasn't visited by the ghosts of fat guys past. Nothing like that but the swelling of my legs and ankles, the stiffness in my joints, the laboring and heavy breathing to do anything were signs that it was giving up. Yes, I have been disabled for three years, yes, I should have started doing this three years ago, No I wasn't in my right mind thru all the changes I had to deal with but like I said earlier it takes a life change sometimes to motivate us to make a change. My sister buying this house in Vegas and asking me to come spend the summer with her. Having an understanding wife that knew I needed to do this and committing 100% to being successful made this all possible. Like I said divine intervention. I hate to regress but there is another trait that most fat people do and that is not read pretty much anything, so for those of you that skipped to this part, you're going to be lost. So here I am in Vegas on Tuesday afternoon June 21ˢᵗ 2016 first things first we unpack and survey the property. Her house is 257 steps from the fitness center and 287 steps to the pool and hot tub. You may be asking yourself why does he know how many step this is? Four days into my journey I purchased a Garmin Vivofit watch. This little device has basically controlled my life since I put it on my wrist. I consider this my tether for fat camp it knows when I've been sleeping it knows when I'm awake it knows when I've been bad and good you get the jest. The Garmin is synced to my phone and my laptop so I always know where I stand on my work outs. I'm getting ahead of myself, I need to back up. So, I wasted no time getting started with my workouts, bright and early Wednesday morning at 5:30 am I hit the pool for round one.

The first day I pretty much swam all of my workouts, I spent four hours in the pool day one. Therefore, I love the pool and why I suggest to every stroke survivor to get in the pool. I don't know of any other workout that you can do on your first day for four hours and other than fatigue not have any other adverse effects from it. Another major change that I implemented at fat camp was eliminating soda and sweets from my diet. So, what you may think, if I died today I probably would have averaged a case of pop a day for my entire life. This is something that I am not proud of and if I play the blame game, this is a product of growing up in the restaurant world. We never drank water at the restaurant you always had a pop and it was like a chain smoker, you seemed to always be refilling the glass before the ice melted. As far as sweets this is a guilty pleasure that I felt I needed to sacrifice for everyone that is sacrificing for me to be out here in fat camp. Both items are a choice no one said you can't have them, this is something that I have chosen to give up there is a difference. When I don't see these items as a need any more I may allow myself to have them again someday. Before I move on from the pop issue here are some thoughts to ponder. Soda holds no nutritional value whatsoever; besides the ungodly amount of sugar it contains it makes up for it with acid, the biggest misconception people on diets believe is that diet soda is better for you because it has no calories. What they fail to realize it the sodium content is far worse for them then the calorie count. So here I am in fat camp, working my way thru my workouts, it is now day four and my nephew and niece purchase me that Garmin I told you about. This was a game changer, here's why. I have stated several times this was a self-imposed fat camp. No one forced me to do anything, my family loves me and have been very supportive. I have basically done this journey on my own though. I get myself out of bed in the morning, I prepare my own meals, I set my work out plans and I do the work outs. My Garmin is like my personal assistant though. The Garmin tracks my footsteps, my calories burnt, my distance traveled and tracks my step challenge's. Challenges you ask? Yep the Garmin has a network of people all over the world that enter these challenges also to motivate them also to push themselves to achieve set goals. Being the competitor I am I can't pass up a good challenge, so every week I push myself to go beyond what I had planned to do, so I can keep my winning streak alive. I have been in three challenges to date and I have won them all. Each week the number increases, I am currently in the 175K challenge, to date I am 11,000 steps shy of a million steps taken since acquiring my Garmin. I have a 54,000-step lead in week four's challenge on my way to four wins in a row. Not bad for a 50-year-old fat guy stroke survivor. I wouldn't think the athletes that I am beating on a weekly basis are too happy with me. I have increased my workout schedule to four times a day. Did I happen to mention that the weather here in Vegas has been above average also. Our average temperature since I have been here being 110 degrees. The standard joke out here is it's a dry heat. I don't care what they say it's frickin hot!!

Either you're in or out: Let me set the record straight, right now!! This is not a diet; one would argue that it's not a weight loss program. This is a lifestyle change motivated by a life changing event. I don't care how much you love a fat person, you can't make them lose weight, if they are not 100% committed to losing the weight. Sure, you can ask them, you can plead with them, show them all the data you want, even threaten to leave them. They may go thru the motions for you and half ass try for you, but they will not see the results you want. Think about it you want this for them, kudos to you for loving them so much. But until they want it for themselves they won't achieve the results they are looking for. Why we are on the subject let me clarify what this fat camp is. I use the term "FAT CAMP" as a metaphor to lose weight, I identify it as self-imposed, because no one is making me do it. I don't consider it a diet because I don't do anything different food wise then I did before I started the camp. Besides eliminating pop and sweets from my food choices. Could I consume them if I wanted too? I am sure I could but no I don't think I would be as happy with my results to date then not consuming them. I also associate diets with having to change everything you do and eat. Buying special foods and supplements that you normally would buy. I eat normal food by my standards, yes, I may have tweaked things a bit, but everyone customizes to fit their needs. For example, this morning I had peanut butter and jelly on a slim bread multigrain bun toasted. Prior to moving to Henderson, I didn't know they existed, my brother in law liked them so I tried it. Bread is bread kind of read the labels fat people you would be amazed how many more calories there are in the exact same items. FAT CAMP TIP. Forever I have always had to have two sandwiches; it didn't matter if I was hungry or not and I don't know if I associated it with being a grown ass man or not. But since starting camp I use one roll, toast both halves, put peanut butter and jelly on both halves and not stick it together. Put them both on the plate and eat them separately. I know it sounds silly but I still get the satisfaction of eating two sandwiches but only get the calories of eating one sandwich. So, I mentioned that I do a smoothie after my morning workout. I use a whey protein powder in the smoothie with my fruit and almond milk. I am not sure if it has any effect on my muscle recovery or not but my muscles don't hurt and I work out every day so you tell me. I also started taking a multivitamin, when I started camp, I believe it is the first time in my adult life that I have ever finished a bottle of vitamins without throwing them away because I stopped taking them. I started taking Glucosamine and Chondroitin tablets three weeks into my workouts to help with joint pain. I have had joint pain for years I figured I would give it a shot and it seems to be working. This also was a choice of mine to start taking them it wasn't a prescribed medication a doctor said I had to take for results. Here was an issue that developed in week four, I told you I was living with my sister in her new place. I was helping her around the house and irritated the muscles in my upper back between my shoulder blades. It really affected my upper body workouts as well as my land walks. I contacted my doctor back in Michigan and told her my situation, she prescribed me Flexeril which is a muscle relaxer that I have used in the past. I did the trick and got me on track in five days but it made me super tired. I slept the most I have slept in years that week. It definitely messed with my schedule, so you need to be flexible but diligent just the same. As far as dinners, portion control is the key here. I allow myself to eat one of whatever we are having. One steak, one chop, one burger on different nights just in case you were getting too excited. A vegetable, potato and we usually have salad. If I am not hungry I take less, what a concept right? Don't heap your plate, remember you are in a partnership with your body. If you cram your pie hole full of food your brain is going to say, hey fat ass why did you have me sweating all day in the pool if you're going to blow it at the table. I am diligent about drinking a glass of water just prior to dinner. Within five minutes up to the time you start eating, any sooner than five minutes your body my start processing the water into your system and out of your stomach. The idea is to fill your stomach with a glass of water that has no calories so you won't be as hungry when you start to eat. I also started drinking water with dinner to keep that idea going thru dinner. Another sight trick I started using was eliminating the salad bowl from the table and putting the salad right on my dinner plate, this way you can fill your plate with salad and it looks like you have a ton of food on your plate, but it is healthy food. Lol You can also use a flavored water to curve cravings when you're really not hungry but you think you are. Raw unsalted almonds, about enough of the palm of your hand is a snack that is actually good for you as well as fruit, any fruit. BS time!!! remember I am not a dietitian but I am still calling BS on this one. Some diets tell you to limit your fruits and vegetable because of the natural sugar and starches in them. This is where I call BULL SHIT!!! I eat as much raw fruit and vegetables as I want. No this doesn't mean that you can open a huge can of fruit cocktail and ladle it down your gully. That is a processed product with preservatives. But if you cut up raw fruit and mixed it together and ate as much as you wanted, more power to you. Fat camp question campers, how many of you have over eaten too much fruit? What typically happens? You shit your brains, out right? This is your body telling you that you overdid it and it's making you pay for it by sitting on the toilet forever it seems. The positive takeaways from this experiment is that you ate a healthy menu item and your body eliminated most of it and anything else in your colon at that time, so you probably lost weight doing it. The same holds true for vegetable, too much and your butt turns into a salad shooter. The other thing to beware of with vegetables is putting outside ingredients on God's creation. If God intended vegetables to taste like Ranch dressing, they would come out of ground tasting like Ranch. Everything in moderation, maybe try vinegar and oil on them. Just a thought, but who am I to tell you how to eat your food. This is your life make your own choices. Portion control is the biggest thing I have done when it comes to my food choices. Yes, I eliminated pop and sweets, but I didn't need them in the first place, they were just empty calories. Yes, they taste good but so does steak and chicken and ribs. I would much rather eat food with taste and substance than useless ones. Water is another key ingredient to success, staying hydrated keeps your muscles going and your body flushing the toxins. Drink as much water as your body needs, I have heard in the past six to eight glasses a day is sufficient. I learned today a gallon of water weighs eight pounds. I do not recommend drinking a gallon of water, but if you live in a hot dry climate drink as much as your body will tolerate. If you are like me maybe water doesn't quench your thirst all the time and you need something with flavor. There are plenty of items on the market that you can add to your water that will give it flavor. Beware of the artificial sweeteners they may using in that product. Some sweeteners can actually make you thirstier than you were in the first place or have a bad aftertaste. Here is a simple and healthy alternative, fill a pitcher with water drop a couple of orange or lemon slices in it, or maybe try putting cucumber or strawberries in it. Place it in your refrigerator and try that for a change. It is a great alternative. Sometimes you're working out hard and your body is telling you that it needs more nutrients. Gatorade and PowerAde are great options to replace electrolytes but they are high in calories, why not try dumping half the bottle of Gatorade in your water bottle and fill the rest of the bottle up with water. It is half the calories and adds some nutrients back into your body. Yes, it doesn't taste the same, but there is value to trying it. Worse case drink the full Gatorade during your workout. You have earned it; you are the one sweating your ass off enjoy!!!

Divine Intervention: So, this is not the part where I give you the Jesus speech or show up on your doorstep with a bible. BUT, I was raised Catholic, I try my best to be a practicing Catholic but sometimes God has me shaking my head. I know we are not suppose too question why God does what he does but the American Way always needs a logical reason for everything. So here I am 48 years old with a brain tumor that needs to be removed. I weighed about 378 lbs. they put me on blood pressure medication about 12 days before surgery. We never discussed this plan B scenario, what if things went wrong? You know reasonable things, everyone just kept saying you will be fine. So, I live thru the 11 ½ hour surgery on the way from surgery to recovery I have a stroke. I wake up basically five days later to the news life as I know it is over. I have paralysis on my left side, I have balance issues and I have very little peripheral vision. I spend almost a month in the hospital. They release me two days before Christmas with a walker and I begin three years of therapy at a local facility. What would you do? I mentioned earlier about the stages of grief, right? Why me? Why now? What am I going to do? Without going dark on you, yes, I contemplated suicide many times. I rationalized, I ran the numbers, I asked God for direction, everything. I concluded that I wasn't brave enough to commit suicide. Brave you say isn't that the easy way out? No, in some cases that's the bravest thing a person can do. I was looking at a dead end, years of therapy. Everything I worked too build was crumbling in front of me. Debt was building and me with no way to take care of any of it. I asked several times, God what is your plan for me? Oh, I forgot to add I am now deaf in my left ear, so maybe God was talking into my bad ear. I have always been a public servant. I have worked in the customer service world forever. I have had the privilege to work with thousands of kids in a school and athletic setting. When I had the opportunity to embark on this unexpected journey I think God has finally decided to give me my mission. There is no logical explanation why now after all that has happened in my life that I would choose to get healthy. Certainly, I should have started this task at a much younger age. Hell, if I would have done it 10 years ago, I would have been 100lbs lighter to start with. The part I have to remember is after I lose this first 100lbs I will still weigh 300 lbs. so I will still be morbidly obese. My goal then will to be lose another 100 lbs. and even at 200 lbs. I will still be morbidly obese. That brings me to the biggest fattest message of all at FAT CAMP. Weight loss is a lifelong journey; it is a marathon not a sprint. Most diet plans are great kick starts to put you on a path but most of us are in such an instant gratification mode, that we want to be done when we first start. It took me 51 years to get to this part of my life. Thru God's grace I hope to spend the rest of my life aking up for my mistakes in the past and get healthier as I do it.

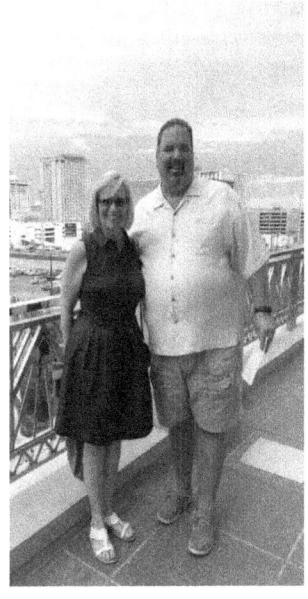 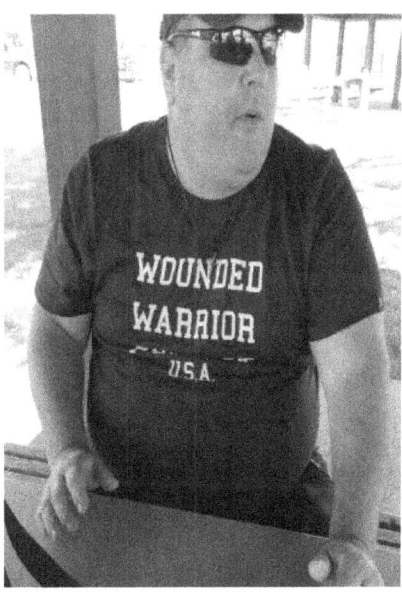 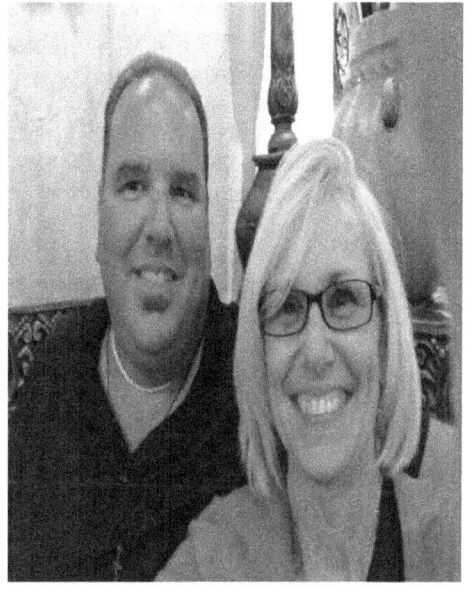

Aren't we all winners: We live in a world today where everyone's a winner, and everyone gets a trophy and everyone goes out for ice cream after the game because we don't keep score anymore because we don't want to hurt anyone's feelings. Sound familiar? Makes me want to puke!!! We live at the fattest era in the history of our country and it's OK with pretty much everyone. Remember when I mentioned that either you're in or out? This is why. There are diet clubs out there that rah rah you into losing weight. Create friendly competitions to encourage you to do your best and as long as you don't beat me everything is great Right. Even the Biggest Loser takes groups of fat people and transforms them into normal sized people with the use of huge amounts of TV show cash and sponsors to pay for everything. These contestants work their asses off for a chance at a big payday if they win. No I don't watch the show that often, but have you ever seen the runner up on the show shed a tear of happiness for completing such a life changing journey? I don't think so, they lost the challenge so they don't get the cash that's all that matters, right? If you ask most fat people, why they want to lose weight. I wouldn't be too surprised to hear them say for acceptance. Time for another BS Call. I hate to burst your bubble but if the group you are trying to fit in with doesn't accept you now the way you are. There is a good fat chance they are not going to accept you when their size. In the long run, you are better off without them. If they are that shallow what good are they. Lose your weight for you, be happy for yourself, your new friends never need to know your past, remember you can't change your past but you can control your future!!

Reboot your system: Have you ever tried rebooting your system? It may be time to do so. Remember when I said we live in a man's world and that we do things the same way always because this is the way we have done it forever? This is your life; this is your journey take control of it. Before I get into my rant remember I am a 51-year-old disabled fat stroke survivor. I have all the time in the world to take this journey, you may not be as fortunate as I am when it comes to time constraints. My BS call on you is that for every excuse you make for not having time to do this. I only need one response to all of them. The most important person in the whole wide world is you and you hardly even know you!! Before you say to yourself I have heard that before, if you are a child of the sixties like I am, think back to Saturday morning cartoons. That was a jingle that one of the School House Rock infomercials used to play way back in the seventies and how relevant is that same message to most of us today. Yes, we are out of tune with our bodies but how do we get back in tune. What do we do when our computer starts working slow or gets a lot of error messages? We reboot it right and most of the time it does the trick. What happens if we ignore the problem? Most of the time the computer crashes. Same thing our bodies do, if we ignore what it is telling us long enough, it crashes and depends on how big the issue is that we ignore. If we ignore our hunger our body reacts with fatigue, weakness maybe headaches. If we ignore sleep, we get sluggish, weakened immunity maybe get sick. When you ignore being fat the price of poker just went up, Diabetes, heart attack, stroke, death. But if you're like me, so it's not going to happen to me I'm invincible, Right!!WRONG!!! There are several products on the market that you can use to cleanse your body and help the rebooting process. For me I didn't use any of them. I did it the old-fashioned way. I started listening to my body. I fed it when it was hungry, I let it sleep whenever it was tired. I gave it extra nutrients to help it fix itself and it rewarded me by letting me continue my incredible journey. I have no other scientific or rational reason other than divine intervention how a 400lb, 51-year-old, stroke survivor could exercise and lose the amount of weight that I have lost in a short time. I am a firm believer that you have to be in tune with your body to get these results.Fat Camp lesson learned August 10, 2016. Case in point, Tuesday night is poker night at the clubhouse on property, I was already tired when I got there, I ignored my body earlier when it wanted to nap. So, poker ran a little long, I got home about 11:30pm I had to catch the Olympic recap and I went to bed about 12:30 am. I set my alarm for 5:30am and quickly fell asleep, so 5:30 the alarm goes off, I roll over and shut it off and attempt to get out of bed. That is when my body yelled Bull Shit!! there was no way it was getting up, so I listened to my body and went back to sleep for another hour and woke up on my own at 6:30 am. We got dressed, I took the long way to the hot tub, spent 10 mins. in the hot tub and proceeded to spend the next five hours and 15 mins. In the pool. I did my lengths, swam 20 laps, and did my lower body workout. Hit the hot tub for 10 more mins. Took the long way home, synced my Garmin when I got home at 40, 047 steps for the morning and started writing. Moral of the story don't fight with your body, listen to it, give it what it needs and it will amaze you with what it will do for you. Piss it off and go pick out your plot…

It's your body: Your body is one of God's greatest creations. Again, I am not trying to force my religious beliefs on anyone. Believe what you want but since this is my journey, this is my interpretation. Our bodies are made up or millions of cells, bones, muscles, ligaments and so on and so on and so on. To me fat is controlled by them all. Your brain is the processor or computer that sends signals to every part of the body. This is where the establishment lives that decides what happens in your body. Its best friend is your heart. They have a mutual agreement they both know they can't live without each other. It's kind of like a marriage when they work together everything is great, but when one of them is not happy neither of them are happy. The brain is the rational side of the relationship the heart tells you what food you like and what food you love. From there you have the blood that that knows both the heart and the brain need blood to survive but it really doesn't care about that because it is too busy to care it's always on the move. Then we have the muscles, the muscles have to listen to the brain, to get directions, it has to be friendly with the blood also because it needs it too. The heart loves the muscles because the harder they work the more blood that flows thru it. You may be thinking by now why is he giving me an anatomy lesson. Listen fat ass get to the point, Right!!! I am, just below the heart especially for fat people because our stomachs are so big is the stomach. Our stomachs have not always been this big, but the more we have eaten over the years have stretched it to this size. Think about it, when it was smaller your body could manage the food intake much faster than when it got huge. The stomach processes the food you eat; the good stuff gets broken down and shipped off to the parts of the body that needs it. The food your body needs gets shipped south, down to the colon awaiting the dump. That could be where the phrase "I got to take a dump comes from." Hey fat guy the point please!!! Getting warmer, just below the stomach in my opinion is the root of all evil!! The genitalia, these two body parts in conjunction with body parts attached to them are a direct correlation with many of our problems. Stay with me here, you can call BS at any time. For a man, most of them are blessed with two heads, more times than not we think with the little one. Men are a simple creature, we could pretty much be happy with sex, food, beer, and money. Not always in that order, it depends on the day but let's call this our NEEDS LIST!!! that brings me to the more complicated member of the food chain, the woman. The woman only has one head that is a good reason why women are more intelligent than men. We have to share time between heads. LOL Women also have a body part that a man spends nine months of his life trying to get out of and the rest of his life trying to get back into. Can I get an Amen? Women know this and they can use it to their advantage and trust me they do. Here though is another one of God's cruel jokes Women can control men pretty much with their vaginas. Remember that is one of man's guilty pleasures. The sick joke is pregnancy!!! Now wait to hear the end of my message before you start chanting kill the fat guy!!! I said nothing about the end product of pregnancy and the joy of birth and the life altering affect a newborn can bring to a family. I am talking about the weight gain, physical changes to the body. Stretch marks, postpartum depression, all of it. Women men did this to you, so any time you withheld sex from us, you are welcome!!! I know this is not funny and for some of us this could be where our downward spiral started. Unless you are one of these overachieving skinny people that should be scared of being eaten by a fat person. You know the ones that have a baby and a week later weight less than before they got pregnant. But I am sure to them they were blimps when they were pregnant, because they were living in our world for nine months. Women don't think that you cornered the market when it comes to baby fat. Men gain weight also during childbearing. Remember most women don't have the same sexual appetite as men do in the first place, now add in weight gain, heartburn, hemorrhoids, raging hormones, and general changes in the body kind of affect the mood. Can I get a hallelujah Mom's!!! this doesn't change the fact that men need sex to stay happy. So entourn men rely on their other guilty pleasures to get us thru those nine months too, food, beer, and money to buy porn so we can take matters into our own hands. LOL It's an ugly cycle now times that by the amount of kids you have and am I on the mark? So now you might be asking OK so now that we are past the child birthing years, why ain't I getting it now? Most fat women don't feel sexy in their current state and when was the last time you told them how beautiful they really are, saying I don't care how big you are, I still love you, isn't the same as saying how beautiful they are. Also, men don't forget you made them this way, you contributed to the process no matter how short of a time it took, Remember the part where I said we gained weight too. Please come lay naked on me and sweat on me with your 400lb body, said no woman EVER!!!

Vivofit My Hero!!! So, I thought I put a section in the book highlighting my Garmin, but apparently, I just talk about it a lot throughout the book. I have to give credit where credit is due, so here you go Garmin, My Garmin changed my life!!! For any of you that saw the movie Castaway with Tom Hanks, my Garmin is my Wilson. It pretty much is my wingman, through all of my fitness trials and decisions. You need to remember for about three months I spent nearly 500 hours virtually alone in workout mode. Yes, on occasion I had interaction with friends, but for the most part, I was alone with my watch, telling me keep going fat ass, more steps needed!! Yes, I am exaggerating the fat ass part is correct but the watch doesn't talk. When the first thing you do in the morning is look at your watch to see what mysterious movements it recorded while you were sleeping. To the last thing, you do at night making sure you synced so you get all your steps for the day and every time you sync during the day as well as looking at the sleep chart to see how long you slept and well as how deep your sleep got. To the miles logged and the calories burnt. Then there are the challenges that keep you moving even when you want to be done. The list goes on and on. Probably the biggest motivation I got from it was from some of the connections I made from people all over the world. I was a legend in my own mind there for a bit when I won eight challenges in a row and the service tech I spoke to from Garmin knew me from my screen name because I had kicked his butt the last four weeks in challenges. The week I was traveling back to Michigan I got a couple messages from Garmin and my connections asking if everything was ok, because they noticed my numbers were down. I thought that was pretty cool. If you need a little extra encouragement, I would totally recommend this product. On a side note, be sure to get the Vivofit 2 or 3 though because they are waterproof up to five meters. I figured if for some reason, I find myself more than 15 feet underwater, the watches problems are the least of my concerns at that point. Lol Here are just a few of the stats I compiled while being on my journey in Vegas

Garmin Steps by day in Vegas.

Day one 6/28/2016:	7/22 29271	8/15 51303	
6/28 3876	7/23 40439 *	8/16 37438	9/8 94100
6/29 8152	7/24 37136	8/17 22807	9/9 72006
6/30 7312	7/25 28289	8/18 41554	9/10 71476
7/1 8941	7/26 23094	8/19 41179	9/11 71728
7/2 11101	7/27 17363	8/20 65056 *	9/12 63612
7/3 11738	7/28 32664	8/21 60062	9/13 84096
7/4 16284 4th of July	7/29 40571	8/22 63245	9/14 55111
7/5 8820	7/30 30774	8/23 50111	9/15 64917
7/6 10846	7/31 31272	8/24 63034	9/16 22631
7/7 17891	8/1 31228	8/25 63482	9/17 54151
7/8 14076	8/2 19063	8/26 62454	9/18 11774 Left for MI
7/9 17519	8/3 24139	8/27 49451	
7/10 13443	8/4 40847	8/28 67932 Birthday	* Depict personal bests
7/11 17569	8/5 44150	8/29 61009	
7/12 15797	8/6 41124	8/30 36122	
7/13 15998	8/7 41127	8/31 61067	
7/14 27063	8/8 40498	9/1 77199 *	
7/15 26085	8/9 33094	9/2 92219 *	
7/16 26015	8/10 24527	9/3 90058	
7/17 22092	8/11 40679	9/4 121863 *	
7/19 18032	8/12 41452	9/5 105445 Labor Day	
7/20 23023	8/13 43124	9/6 78153	
7/21 26059	8/14 50164 *	9/7 100085	

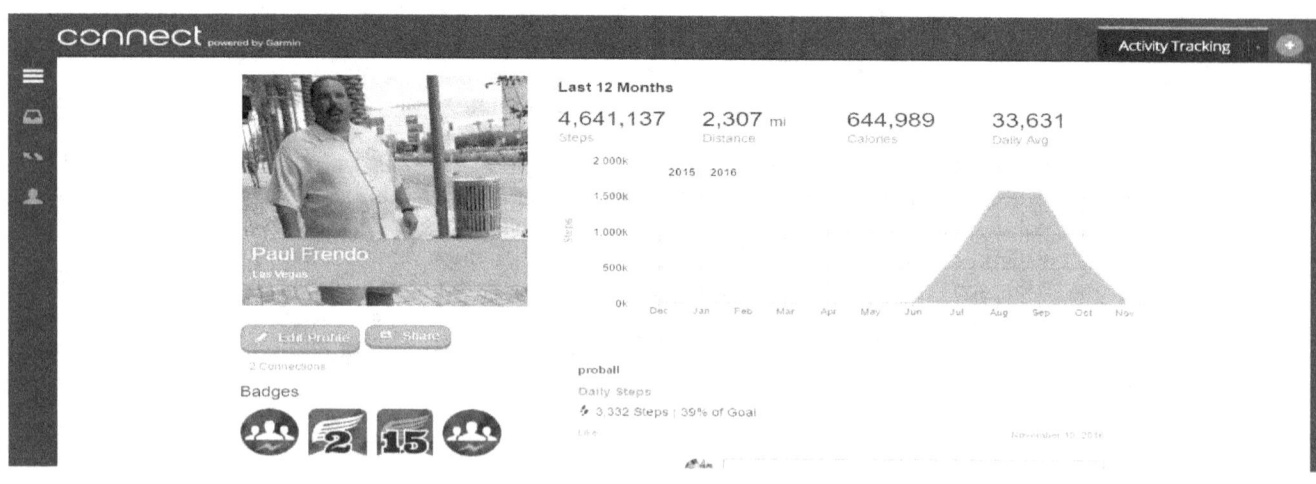

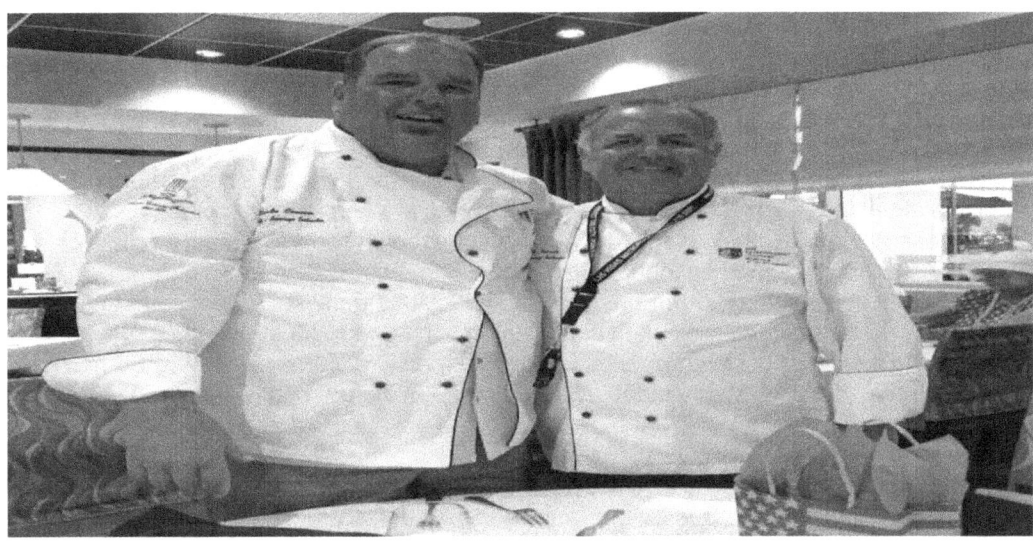

Chef for a day!! Have you ever had someone make you feel so special that you felt like a king or a queen for a day. Well that happened to me and it was freaking awesome. I have talked about Chef Claude on more than one occasion throughout the book. Chef Claude has lived a very exciting and memorable life as a chef. He has been the executive chef to Steve Wynn at his Casino's in Vegas as well as the Executive Chef at Harrah's in London. He recently retired from the Las Vegas Institute of Arts, where he was the Director of the Culinary Program. A group of us had the privilege to attend one of his last dinner services at the school. We surprised him by bringing his wife along with us and presented him with his own Garmin as a retirement gift. Chef Claude pulled out all the stops for us. He and his staff prepared an exquisite meal as well as Champagne and wine. He even took time out of his busy evening to play the piano for us, beautifully I must add. Just when I thought the wonderful night was over. Chef Claude honored me with one of his chef coats signed "to Paul, the most committed. Claude." It meant the world to me, I have always considered myself capable in the kitchen, but to have a Chef as experienced as Chef Claude recognize me for my dedication to fitness and nutrition, blew me away. It is definitely a night I will long remember and I am sure all my friends that attended the evening shared in that experience as well. Not to mention that the coat I am wearing in the picture is a XL. That is the first XL I have worn in years. Most of the clothes I packed for Vegas were 4XL. Chef Claude and I shared many morning walks the last month I was at the Villa's. He had started his own journey to lose 15 lbs. by the time he left for France at the end of September. I got a message from him today, that he has lost 10 lbs. so far with a week to go. I wish him all the best on his journey. In our many talks, we had throughout the days, Claude told me the story of why he decided to be a chef. Claude grew up in France as a child, his family didn't have a lot of money, so as the oldest boy in the family he helped out his father delivering mushrooms to the local restaurants. Most of the time this was late at night. He explained to me one cold night he stopped in front of one of the restaurants they delivered to and he watched the chefs feverishly prepare the food for their customers. One of the chef's noticed Claude watching and knew it had to be cold out there, so he prepared Claude what would be equivalent to one of our Chicago style hot dogs. Claude said it was the best hot dog he ever had and from that day forward he wanted to become a chef. Low and behold all his hard work paid off and he became one of the top chef's in the business. It just proves that hard work and a great work ethic can do great things

Scale this!!! Fat Camp rule: I hate scales, the only reason I use one is to document my weight loss journey. Other than that, I despise them. A person should base the success of their journey on how they feel and how their clothes fit. One of the biggest traps we fall into and probably the biggest killer of most diets is that muscle weighs more than fat. So, you work your ass off for a week, you stick to your diet and you make it to weigh in day, you strip down because you know your cloths add 20 pounds to you, right. You step on the scale and see no loss and God forbid you see a gain because that's when you go from one scale to a ton of pieces of a scale. Some people even weigh themselves daily. How crazy is that. Did you know a gallon of water weighs eight pounds? So, if you are drinking a lot of water, you still gain weight while your body processes that water and you eliminate it from your system. Second, muscle weighs more than fat, just because you are just walking in the water, you are still converting fat to muscle and the muscles you are using to walk are filling with blood as you use them so that's why you gain initially. Case in point, I am in week four of my journey, the prior week I lost six pounds, I had logged 101,000 steps that week. Week four I logged 200,600 steps and that was the week my back spasms started so I didn't go to the gym at all that week I just worked in the pool and walked some on land. So, I get to Monday morning excited to step on the scale and see the progress I have made. Guess how happy I was to find out I didn't lose anything, not even an ounce I was the exact same weight. If I didn't feel better, and was still buzzing since I won my second Garmin challenge, I could have easily lost focus. My sister pointed out the fact that at least you didn't gain anything. It didn't help my state of mind at the time, but it did add fuel to my fire to work harder in week five. In week five I logged 253,000 steps and won my fourth Garmin challenge and weighted in seven pounds lighter. So, persistence paid off there So here is the skinny on why I don't have an official start weight. When I arrived at Henderson (Fat Camp) upon surveying the facilities. I came across this ugly, white, fairly unused POS piece of equipment sitting in the corner of the fitness facility. Yes, for you skinny people it's your daily affirmation tool that tells you that you are still skinny, but for a fat SOB such as myself it's the devil. A SCALE, except this devil was even a more evil one than usual. It only went up to 300 on the main weights I don't remember how much the slide bar counted, all I know is I was pisssssssssed off, because it wouldn't register my weight in the beginning. That bastard just sat in the corner staring at me as to say na na na boo boo, do another set fat ass, you're never gonna step on me. So, I used that as motivation, I never did step on it when I was under it's pathetic weight requirements. Not to say I didn't kick it a couple times in passing, but no blood no foul right!! One morning in week two of camp I was cleaning the grout in my sister's bathroom and discovered she had a digital scale in there that went up to 400 lbs. The first time I stepped on it, I heard it say GET OFF!!! And the scary part about that was it didn't have a speaker that I knew of. LOL After that we became friends and as I lost weight it seemed to like me even more and we lived happily ever after, the end. NOT!!! So, I am home here in Michigan and I am trying to get back in sync with my weight loss, Hence the word trying, let's just say there is an adjustment period. Trying to get caught up on being gone for three months, catching up on doctor's appointments, reestablishing physical therapy, getting re-signed up for the gym. You know the usual crap that keeps us from working out in the first place. I must tell you I sweat more yesterday carrying a weed whip around the yard then I sweat total at fat camp and we are only talking about two hours of weed whipping. Go figure. Physical Therapy? I will come back to that; I have to finish my scale story before I forget my point. So, Monday's is my day to weigh in, right? Before I left for Vegas, we had our own digital scale. Apparently, my daughter decided she wanted a different scale and tossed the old one and purchased a scale with the weight dial on it and son of a bitch if the scale tops out at 280 lbs. I want to stay in good graces with this one, so I didn't even waste my time shocking it with my fat ass jumping on it and try to play the addition guess the weight game when the big hand passes the max weight and heads into no man's land on its second time around. I figured I would make friends with the one at the fitness center, the twin of the bitch back in Henderson, I think I will call this one the wicked witch of the East. If she doesn't come up with the numbers I am looking to achieve then I will drop a house on her ass. Lol Now back to reality, physical therapy. Yep throughout this journey I have still been disabled. I suffer from many things related to the stroke and being fat of course. Probably one of the biggest recurring problems associated with the stroke has been lack of range of motion in my neck. Remember I am not a doctor; all I know is what I hear from doctors and what I read on the internet. From what I can surmise, during my stroke I had a brain herniation, residual effects from the herniation is progressive loss in range of motion in your neck. The only thing that seems to help my neck stay flexible is manipulation that I receive at PT, so other than maybe having my neck fused or something stupid like that PT is my best option. So yes, that's why I still go to PT nearly three years after my stroke and up to three times a week.

Got a pill for that? Thank you too big pharm, for inventing a pill for everything. Again, before the chanting begins there are definitely medications out there that are a necessity for some of us to survive on. Especially after we have abused our bodies for so long. I still have to take five blood pressure pills a day till I see my family doctor when I get back to Michigan. I am working towards the day I can be medication free. As my good buddy, Jack used to always say, "someday but not today! "This brings me to my next ah ha moment. Hospitals scare the hell out of me. If you need any more motivation then you already have, go into the hospital. Let me preface this rant by first saying the nurses and staff that took care of me at Blodgett and Mary Free Bed. Did an excellent job, I owe them my life? For others, though, the hospital is not where you want to be. The longer you stay in the hospital the less of a chance you have of ever getting out. Think about it you are surrounded by sick people, germs, viruses, and let's not even go to the food there. They wake you up to make sure you are sleeping you are on their schedule, based on their shifts and their rules. I have been self-employed as much as I have been employed in corporate America over my lifetime. Whenever I was asked by a doctor how I was doing, my standard answer was good, remember I was living in their world. I knew if I told them about my vision problems, balance issues and headaches, I wasn't getting out of there anytime soon. I beat the odds to recovering from the stroke I had and to think my size played a major factor for the stroke in the first place. I am not trying to scare you with horror stories of my fun in the hospital but it would be a disservice to you if I didn't tell you about it.

Healthy Restaurant Choices: What's wrong with this picture? If you loved my rant about hospitals you're going to love this one. Restaurants are the worst thing that ever happened to the fight against fatness. First things first, you notice I didn't use the word all, but unless that restaurant grows all their own vegetables in their back yards and raises their own meats and poultry and catches their own fish it will never be as good for you as home cooking. It's not their fault completely, they have to deal with the FDA as well as their local health departments to make sure you don't die from any one of the many foodborne illnesses out there. So, in order to help limit the risk to you, extra preservatives, more frozen foods are used, higher cooking temps are used and more seasonings are used to bring the food back to life so it is edible. Now add in the fact that we are such an impatient society. We want it fast and we want to eat it even faster so we can be back to our fast-paced life, Right? I have already talked about making healthy food choices, we think that if we go to a restaurant, even a fast food restaurant and order a salad and wash it down with a supersized diet soda, we are on the right track to a healthy lifestyle. It's a start of something, but why subject yourself to the temptation. Does this sound familiar, I just ate a salad and saved on calories I can treat myself to a little dessert. Right? Been there done that. Again, restaurants spend billions of dollars a year on advertising, telling you what you want to hear, healthy choices, health smart, weight watchers approved. As a thirty-year veteran of the restaurant industry, every meal you can make at home is the healthiest meal choice you can make. Again, I am not saying all, so put your knives and forks down and back away from the skinny person. The industry in a whole has tried to get healthier, but remember safety first, if you make it through the meal and live too come back for more, they win right. Life story, I owned a couple of fast food restaurants back in my 20's. I had a friend that I graduated high school with, frequent my establishment quite a bit. He was a fat guy like me but he also had a thyroid issue that he never could get under control. He ended up dyeing before our 10-year reunion, he weighed over 500 pounds at the time of his death. We played football together and at one time we both were under 200 lbs. That's how quickly the weight can balloon on you. I felt guilty for a long time after his death, I felt that I contributed in some way because he liked my food. But food is an addiction if he didn't get it from me, he would have gotten it from someone else. RIP Jeff, 78 forever.

ADDICTED!!! Food is a drug to fat people. Our body always craves it; you can go thru withdrawals. It affects your moods when you don't get it. It will drive some people to even steal it if they can't afford to pay for it. Why hasn't some government agency ever looked into the adverse effects food have on people? Easy food consumption doesn't affect everyone the same way. So, what my body hoards your body might let it pass thru you. You ever have a friend or even a family member that had such a high metabolism that they could literally eat more food than you and him/her and never gain an ounce. Another one of God's cruel jokes. That is why I preach portion control and menu exploration. Try new things, see how they affect your body. If your body is compatible with it keep it or move on. If all else fails do what I do and just burn more calories, than you take in. Life lesson, I mentioned before I trained and coached ball players. I coached a player, one that was a six foot five, a left-handed pitcher that graduated high school at 180 lbs. He got a baseball scholarship to college and the head coach liked his stuff but wanted him to gain 20 lbs. before the season. Six months later after countless trips to the gym and trips to the golden arches, he was cut from the team because the harder he tried to gain the more weight he lost. Boy, I wish I had that problem. You can also get addicted to working out. Many people especially after you see a result can get addicted to working out. I know Claude loved to walk in the pool, he would take every chance he had to walk in the pool. He was up to eight pounds lost before I left. His goal was at least 15 pounds before he went to France by the end of September. You need to know he was only about 185 lbs. so he didn't have as much extra weight as I did. I also tell him how great his progress is. He is a great guy and an awesome chef.

Do it or Diet: Have you ever been or knew of a person that was constantly on a diet? It could always be the same diet, but the results were never what they expected. Some people call them yoyo diets cause their weight goes up and down. Think about it, they probably were working towards something with a deadline. A wedding, reunion, family event but whatever it was they might hit their goal but the weight came right back after the event was over. This ties into my thoughts on making a deal with your body. When you only set goals to meet an event deadline your body may or may not cooperate with you. Yes, you have a better chance of achieving your goal if you work in conjunction with your body through the process of the weight loss, but the minute you stop working together it falls apart. Think about it, women when you are focused on losing weight for a wedding, not only are you looking to fit into a dress. You get to go shopping, get your hair done, maybe a mani & pedi. Maybe even go to the spa to rejuvenate? These are all positive for your psyche Right. You get me in the dress and I will make you look great and it's a self-esteem boost. What do you use as a bargaining chip when you just want to lose weight, most of us use guilty pleasures to get results? The sad part about this practice is that we call it cheating on my diet. You're not cheating on your diet; you are cheating on yourself. See we have been hearing the word diet so long we act like it's a member of the family, like it's one of our lost children. You have been doing it so long it might as well be one. Next time you say I need to go on a diet, you may want to ask yourself why. If the answer is not for you, then you're wasting your time and effort. If you don't buy it, it isn't yours to own. Just a tip.

Love your Kids: Parents, especially parents with fat kids, it is your responsibility to guide your children through the pitfalls of an unhealthy lifestyle. They don't know the dangers of high fructose corn syrup or MSG. they just know that it tastes good or their friends eat it or there is a cool prize in the bottom of the box. Introduce them early in life to all that the food world has to offer them. Give them raw vegetables, spice them up make them fun and if they don't like them the first time don't give up on them. Yes, it is easier to give them what they want, but it's a lot harder for them to go through life as the fat kid and deal with all the health issues they face in the future because of the choices we make as kids. Good eating habits are learned early in life and have a tendency to stay with us for life. I know it is hard to break some of the bad habits we continue to abuse our bodies with on a daily basis. Be diligent and consistent with the messages you tell your kids and I personally feel the do as I say not what I do approach is one of our kids biggest BS calls we never want to admit hearing. Remember we are the adults here, who are they to question what we do? They do because they love us and even though we sometimes think they aren't listening to us they seem to never miss anything. Don't be afraid to add a little something something to their fruits and veggies if they don't like them raw. Yes, whipped cream adds empty calories but it is still lower in calories than ice cream or cake. We are in the midst of creating generation XXL and they are only getting bigger. We need to break the chain before it breaks us.

The last supper: Time for an ah ha moment, now without getting too religious on you. Fat people treat supper time like it could be their last and it very well might be, Statistics prove that fat people have a shorter life expectancy. Keep on eating the quantity you are and making the food choices you do and continue to build on that statistic or break the mold and work to get healthy and be a success story, the choice is yours. Remember we are not guaranteed tomorrow, yesterday is history, tomorrow is a mystery, today is a present from God. Enjoy your present but don't expect the presents to keep coming unless you are willing to make the changes necessary to be around to enjoy them. Why do we feel the need to eat till we are full? Why can't we just eat till we are satisfied? Challenge yourself to eat what you want but only enough to get a good taste of it. This would be almost like grazing but with a full meal. No, I'm not saying eat like a bird. But here in a concept for you, leave the table hungry if you have to, prove to your body that you mean business. If you don't shake up your body, then why will it think anything is different?

Are you on the juice? In today's world, this could be such a hot button. No I am not talking about steroids. I am talking about fruit or vegetable juice and all the natural benefits from juicing. I watched a documentary recently by Joe Cross from Australia on his journey to a healthier life by going totally juice as his diet. I have to admit that I am a bit skeptical on non-protein diet plans. I guess if you were that disciplined to do only juice and could stay on that program until you could break your poor dietary habits it is worth a try. I know for me personally I have failed more than once doing the liquid diets. Sure, the weight comes off quickly but I never did them long enough to learn how to continue on the journey and keep the weight off. In my case the weight came back with a vengeance and I weighed more after my body repaid me for starving it in the first place. The documentary is worth the watch though; it is very inspirational and beneficial and explains the benefits of juicing I recommend watching it. For several weeks, I did a fruit smoothie after my morning workout that consisted of frozen strawberries, banana, whey, almond milk, and blueberries. I also incorporated melons, vegetables, apples, lemons, and limes. Whatever was available at the time. I progressed my beverage selections also. I went from country time lemonade, to natural fruit juices made in the emulsifier. I used agave nectar as a base and added whatever fruit we had available. Most of the time I used watermelon, strawberry, apple, lemon, limes, and banana for sweetness. It tastes delicious the only downside that I found was the longer it sat in the pitcher the more it ferments because the fruits start to meld together and remember there are no preservatives added so the quicker you used the juice the better it tasted. No I am not sure how many calories there was per glass, but I didn't care, it wasn't a can of soda or beer or a processed sugared down fruit juice so like I said I didn't care about the calories. On the subject of hydration, I prefer something more than just water. Don't get me wrong water is you friend but sometimes you need more. I was looking to replace my electrolytes and I found a product that I think worked for me. Emergent-C. I got it in a lemon flavor, it seemed to do the trick I drank one bottle of water mixed with one packet of Emergen-C and I never felt dehydrated or showed any signs of dehydration and remember I spent over 10 hours some days in 115 degree temperatures in that pool. Not sure what I would have felt like without it but I didn't want to find out the hard way. As a longtime coach, if I had a nickel for every time I told one of my players to make sure they stayed hydrated I would have a lot of nickels. The same holds true for us as active exercisers. Give your bodies what it needs and it will do amazing things, deprive it of what it needs and prepare for its wrath. I don't know about you but I prefer to take care of it now and not have to suffer anymore. One the same line as a need for hydration, your body requires protein as fuel to keep going and sustain your energy level. Remember in moderation. You notice I didn't say a full meal!!! I said protein. Peanut butter on thin bread, or a granola bar, maybe a couple scrambled eggs. Not eggs, bacon, sausage, potatoes, pancakes, toast, and juice then plan to go do your work out. You are setting yourself up for disaster and unless you plan to work out on the toilet, that's where you will probably end your workout. Remember you are in a partnership with your body, each part of your body has to contribute for you to be successful. Each part is important but all of them contribute differently, you have to be the coach of your body and get it to work together to keep it in harmony. Remember my breakdown of how the body works? Food and water will make the stomach and muscles happy, sun glasses when the sun is bright will make your eyes happy as well as less strain on the brain. Stretching before you get too far into your workout will also make your muscles happy. Maybe your body prefers not walking during the hottest time of the day. Maybe it's not a morning person, so cut it some slack, let it wake up fully before you decide to push it to the limit. I know you might be calling Bull Shit on me real soon. Listen fat guy, I tell my body when, why and how hard to work. Kudos to you I have learned through my 51 years on this planet that you catch more flies with honey than vinegar. My body works better and harder for me when I started listening to it than it did when I told it what to do. It's your journey, good luck. Humans can learn a lot from animals about weight control. Animals forge all year long and store up food for a long winter to be able to survive. Humans have adapted to their thinking as well as our founding founders since they didn't have preservatives and refrigeration to store food. We are so worried about running out of food or even where or next meal will come from that we are worried that won't be enough food tomorrow so we better eat all we can today. The difference between us, animals and even our forefathers is most of us don't gather, grow, hunt, and prepare our own food. We either buy it from the grocery or a restaurant so we don't burn any calories during the gathering process. Chew on that for a while and see if you fall into that category.

Ready Set Eat!!! I come from a large Maltese family, for those of you that don't know where Malta is my condolences but as my father would always say "Malta is about 100 miles to the good of Italy." So, food was always a priority with us, we learned at an early age that if you wanted to get enough to eat, you better eat fast. On rare occasions my mother would serve a dinner that required the use of a knife, because she wanted to limit the amount of bloodshed from arms reaching across the table and returning back to your body with puncture wounds. Lol I'm exaggerating but not by much. It was pretty much an unwritten rule that you didn't reach too close to any of my sibling's plates for fear of retaliation. My mother felt sorry for my younger sister and I because of the vast age difference between us and my older brothers and sisters so she would usually start the food festivities closer to our end of the table. Then it was everyone for themselves. My father worked late most nights so other than Sunday dinner we didn't have his support to protect us. Not that any of us were dumb enough to not mind my mother, she was wicked with a wooden spoon or God forbid she broke out the fly swatter, that woman had a better whip action on her wrist then most major league pitchers do today. Both my brothers were over six feet and 200 lbs. in middle school, they had the advantage over me because they could make it up the stairs before me in case she grabbed a shoe. She was also more accurate than most MLB pitchers also. My mother was Irish, English, Scottish and she would always throw in Hillbilly since she was raised in the south. She taught me so much about cooking and creating food from leftovers then one deserves to know. Like I said though in my younger days with all the mouths to feed, left overs didn't exist. As I got older and the herd thinned out my mother had issues preparing the proper amount of food for the number of people she had at the dinner table. So, that's where her favorite meal was born "slumgullian" which basically meant anything she had left in the refrigerator that needed to be cooked before it went bad. She figured if she put her spin on it and enough seasonings in it, it would be edible and for the most part she was right. Plus, none of us were stupid enough to question her or pass up dinner, right? My favorite Christmas cookie to this date is my mother's version of a "whatsit" This is the last cookie she would make after baking what seemed to her about 100 dozen cookies for the 11 of us. She would combine all the ingredients she had left over from all the other recipes, put her spin on them, bake them and it was heaven on a cookie sheet to most of us. Not sure what the calorie count was but that is probably, ok most definitely where my lack of concern I foster for calorie intake began.

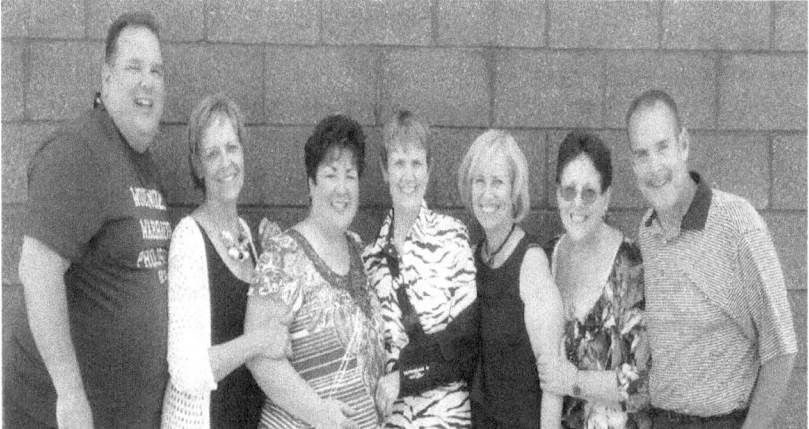

To put things into better perspective on how important food was to us back in my childhood. For as long as I could remember for Thanksgiving my mother used to cook two turkeys that were over 20 lbs. each, stuff them both with an extra pan of stuffing, at least 10 lbs. of mashed potatoes, green bean casserole, corn, dinner rolls, green jello, yams, don't forget the gravy then it was time for pie. Pumpkin, apple, mincemeat, and Cool Whip in a tub and plenty of tubs trust me. It took her most of the week to prepare the feast and pretty much less than 30 minutes for us to devour it. She made the two turkeys so we would have left overs through the weekend. As time went on and more of my siblings left the nest, more and more of the menu items lasted longer through the weekend.

What's for dinner? Being an inquisitive child I always thought of ways to maximize whatever I put my mind to. Dinner time was no different, I think that's why I always asked what's for dinner? So, I could focus on what food to attack food when it was brought to the table. If it was pasta, check steak on rare occasions, check, pizza a no brainer, check then I would pan out to the vegetables and salad. Unfortunately for me my siblings had the same plan of attack, hence the potential bloodshed. So, that began our need for speed, the house rule is that you had to finish what you had on your plate before you had seconds. Seconds on most nights were not an option because they were gone the first time around. I give my mother a world of credit, we were not rich by any means but she always made sure that we all had at least on full plate. I still think this is why to this very day I ask who ever I am eating dinner with "what's for dinner?" Even if I am the one cooking so I can plan my route for dinner. I know I drive my wife

crazy when I always ask her what she wants for dinner. We might have just finished breakfast and I will still ask her what she wants dinner. She doesn't share the same passion I have for food. She came from a smaller family that was not in the restaurant business. Her mother is a very good cook but it wasn't such a cumbersome ordeal for dinner time at her house. I need to prepare, shop, prep and plan out dinner for me to feel good about dinner. That stemmed on of my sister and my biggest arguments over this past summer. I love to cook and take my time to cook it right. She on the other hand is a very impatient cook. She wants it done yesterday, she is a good cook also in her own way. For me good food can't be rushed you need to use the ingredients you cook with to help season the dish you are preparing. If you rush it, you just taste the seasoning you added to the dish and not the dish itself. That's just my opinion I could be wrong. But since this is my journey I am never wrong. Lol

Fill er up!! This brings me to another Ah Ha moment, statistics prove the faster you eat the more you weigh, so why don't we slow down? It is a proven fact that it can take up to 20 minutes for your body to register you are full. I don't know about you but I could finish a small pizza by myself in less than 20 minutes'. Some people use the putting your fork down between bites method to trick your body into eating less. Here is a suggestion how about only taking enough food on your plate that your body needs and not eat any more than that? I know that is easier said than done, but it is possible to do, right? We're not looking for the cure for cancer here. Just looking to shed some pounds and live a healthier lifestyle. Filling your stomach with healthier food choices is a great start. That is why I don't limit myself to how much fruits and vegetables I eat. It beats plugging my pie hole with extra pizza, burgers, or pasta. Listen carefully to your bodies, it will tell you what it needs, even if it is an unhealthy choice. Remember everything in moderation. Take care of your body and it will take care of you. Don't you remember that damn rabbit on the Trix cereal commercials. Trix, Trix are for kids. It's hard to build a harmony with your body if you try to trick it all the time with gimmicks. Try giving it what it needs for a change and ask it to respond in kind.

Leave me alone!! If it was just that easy. Weight loss products are a billion $$ business, if fat people wanted to be left alone they would stop buying these products. I know skinny people make up a good portion of the people buying these products. Nothing insults my ego and intelligent more than seeing a bunch of size 0's sweating to the latest hip hop crap and preaching to me on how they lost 10 pounds sweating off the weight. Don't get me wrong while I still have a pulse in this fat ass body, I won't mind seeing a size 0 in a skin-tight bodysuit with a genetically modified body jump around on my tv screen in front of me. I am a remote control away from a Baywatch moment. I'm calling B.S. to any man out there that says they don't do the same thing. I know you ladies don't feel the same thing when they show the Hofmeister running on the beach. So, if you won't give up on diet products, why do you think they are going to give up on you. Mark my words if some company told you today, take this pill and you would have the body of your dreams. No special diets, no exercise. News flash it's already out there and has been out there for a long time. Why aren't we all skinny then? They DON'T work that's why. Let me back up a bit so I don't get sued by one of them. They don't work. Have you ever heard the word placebo? This is a pill that says this is the results you should experience if you take the pill. If you follow their plan long enough and even though it says no dieting or exercise required most of them still highly suggest for quicker results healthy food choices and living an active lifestyle will enhance the losing process. Am I, right? Been there done that, no loss still fat!! We are so desperate to lose weight without doing it the right way, we will pretty much try anything. I particularly like the products that target belly fat. Hahahahahahahah Doctors are just getting the technology to be able to zip cancer cells without having to flood the entire body with radiation at the low cost of thousands of dollars a visit and we think for one low cost of $9.99 we can lose that stubborn belly fat. Fat chance. I would challenge you that you could lose as much weight as you want for little or no cost to you. Eat healthier, control your portions, and walk as much as possible. The more you do these three things the more weight you will lose. If you don't lose weight what are you out, time? We are all pretty much out of time anyway. Right? It's a sad statistic that most Americans Joe Cross interviewed on his journey across America said that they knew they were morbidly obese he said if he could show them an easy way to lose weight that taste good, would they try it to get healthier and most of them said no. they were to set in their ways or they said they were too old to change or made up even worse excuses not to want to try. Some of them had kids, some were married and some were young but they all had excuses why they wouldn't try. How many people have you known in your lifetime that didn't care how they lived until the doctor gave them a death sentence and then they tried everything they could to try to keep living but still died? So, sad!!!

Break the cycle!! I mentioned earlier in the book that I was blessed with three beautiful children. Each of them share the same dna, but all were born into different stages of my wife and my life journey. My oldest daughter was born into my life of restaurants so unfortunately for her she was raised primarily on fast food, until she was about 8. Shortly after that we moved to Hesperia, MI when my son was in kindergarten and Hesperia is a rural West Michigan Village, with a couple of mom and pop restaurants it does have a subway restaurant now that is the closest thing to fast food that we have within 15 mins. So, my son grew up on a mix of home cooking and fast food. My youngest was almost a year old when we moved. She grew up on a majority of home cooking with a little fast food sprinkled in. Out of the three children my oldest has had the hardest time with her weight. She has to work the hardest of the three to keep her weight under control. My Son was very active with sports that helped him maintain a healthy athletic build. My youngest has been the most adventurous eater of the three she pretty much like most food. She will try anything pretty much once. She still has to watch what she eats or it sticks to her.

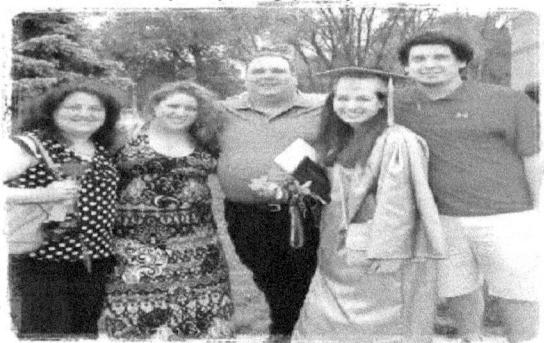 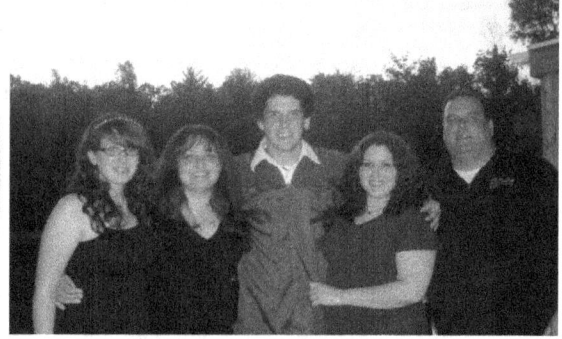

I guess this would be a good time to expand on entire family dynamic. I have eight living brothers and sisters. Five sisters and two brothers. I also have 26 nieces and nephews and I have 19 great nieces and nephews. Of which eight of us struggle with weight issues, three of my siblings have had bariatric surgery. Two of my sisters tested positive for silica's disease. Six of the nieces and nephews have silica's disease and five of my great nieces and nephews have silica's also. So, there is a good chance that silica plays a big part in my children's issues with gluten. All three of my kids deal with acid reflux as well. My son just started living gluten free and is feeling better since switching to this plan. The sister that I spent the summer with is gluten free, so I found myself following her restrictions and I have found myself feeling better. I am going to continue limiting gluten from my menu options as often as possible. It is amazing how the chemicals in foods affect our bodies. I have learned thru my sister's bad experiences how harsh gluten can make her sick. It's time for another B.S. call. Just because a restaurant claims to have gluten free menu choice don't feel safe unless you ask these simple questions. Does the kitchen use separate cooking utensils when preparing their gluten free menu items? If you are eating GF pasta, do they use a separate pot of water that they only cook their GF pasta in? In warm climate states, we found that Mexican Restaurants put flour in their cheese to keep it from clumping, they don't realize that to a gluten free person even though the cheese is an afterthought the flour in that cheese will bring hours if not days of discomfort for that person. If you find yourself getting sick after you eat certain flour or wheat based foods or if you suffer from acid reflux you might want to get tested for silica's.

WWW WTF: We live in such an instant world, coming from a world of news print and television news. Modern communication is incredible. Being a product of the 60's it is hard for the younger generation to relate to people even in their 50's. Growing up I didn't have computers, cell phones, internet and even microwave ovens were not invented when I was in my teens. So, it's harder for us from the older generation to adapt to the new world. Technology is your friend, really… Used correctly it can be a great tool in the fight against fat. My Garmin Vivofit has been a huge motivational tool I constantly check it to see how many steps I have walked on a daily basis. I dropped out of this week's challenge on Tuesday of this week. I was up to the 475,000 challenge and I knew with the three days of travel and getting re acclimated back to Michigan would stress me out enough then to worry about getting 100,000 steps a day. I have found myself not being as motivated since dropping out of the challenge. Getting back to technology, social media can also be a big motivator. Facebook when used correctly can usually generate positive feedback when someone posts something relevant and without overkill. If someone posted that they lost 10 lbs. on their journey that is worth posting. If someone posts I have been dieting for 10 mins and haven't seen any change yet. Not worth the post. All I'm saying is it does a body good when you get positive feedback. Take people on your journey with you, just don't over post your updates, that is the quickest ways to lose friends.

Let's make a deal!! So how many of you like to play "let's make a deal" with anything. If you say not me I call B.S. we do it all the time. Husbands do it to wife, If I get to go golfing then I will come home and take you out to dinner. Win win for us by the way. Wives do it to husbands. Let's go shopping, I don't want to go by myself, there might be a little something something in it for you later. Again, win win. We do it to our kids, get good grades and I will take you out to Chuck E Cheese. We do it to our bodies all the time, get me thru this weekend and I will rest you next week. I know you're hungry but it isn't dinner time yet, just a couple more hours then I will feed you. Every time you make a deal you enter into a trust situation, what happens when you make that deal and don't follow thru with it? So, you have a bad round of golf, you come home and forgot the game was on so you tell your wife sorry honey, the games on can we order a pizza instead. She has spent four hours getting ready, full makeup, changed clothes three times, and even shaved her legs, A, B.S. call is waiting in the wings for any man that thinks ordering pizza delivery will satisfy this situation. Scenario two, your wife drags you thru every store in the mall, you go willingly and don't whine the whole day, you come home, carry all the bags in, she jumps in bed and falls asleep, totally acceptable, Right? Hell, to the no!!!Scenario three your kids bust their butts and get good grades, they expect to see the big rat and play some games, you think if you welch on that promise, you think your kids won't hold that against you for life? Fur sure! So, what makes you think every time we break a promise to our bodies it's not going to get back at you? Sure, go ahead and eat what you want, that's going right to your ass, don't exercise, no problem how about a little heart attack? Keep doing it and how about a dirt nap? Trust issues, live clean and live right and things have a better chance of running better than the alternatives.

Pool Time Fun!!! So, I have explained bits and pieces of what I do in the pool. I have met many people in the pool and out of the pool that want to know how I have lost so much weight. I know many of them have their B.S. card ready and so want to throw it in my face. But after 79 days straight of working out in the pool, I don't think anyone of them still wants to show their card. I leave Vegas 85 lbs. lighter; I leave the casino's a little bit of my money. I leave with a SUV full of treasures hunted on six Saturdays. I leave with fond memories and friendships made that I hope to rekindle again in the near future. I leave with a feeling of satisfaction that I know my hard work has made a difference to me and the many people that I have come in contact with that called me their inspiration to lead a healthier lifestyle and get in shape. I feel that I have accomplished so much in what seems such a little time, but I also have so much more to do. I still have to lose my additional 15 lbs. to reach my 100 lbs. of my first journey. I need to figure out how I want to attack my second 100 lbs. to reach my ultimate goal of 200 lbs. With that goal brings more obstacles that I will need to overcome. Winter in Michigan, the holidays, life in general and most of all the motivation to continue to want to keep losing. I credit my Garmin Vivofit 3 for keeping me on the straight and narrow throughout my journey, I purchased my Garmin on Sunday June 27ᵗʰ 2016 and from the first day I felt compelled to push myself to meet the goal set by my watch. Each week that number grew, day by day week by week the goal increased and the challenges got tougher. I believe the first challenge I competed in was a 35,000-step challenge. The last challenge I won on week nine was 350,000 steps. I had several days that I logged over 100,000 steps for the day. I ended my Vegas journey logging over 3,409,000 steps I walked over 1700 miles burnt over 220,000 calories and averaged 47,000 steps a day. I ended up replacing two watches before getting my final watch. I never thought in a million years I could log the steps and goals I have attained over the journey. I would personally like to thank all the people that spent time developing this product. If you are a person that is technology friendly and need a motivational tool to keep you motivated. I would recommend this wholeheartedly. In conjunction with the walking, I did water resistant work. I rotated my work outs daily between upper and lower body workouts. I guess this would be a good time to clarify what a workout consists of. I try to follow a simple rule that I firmly believe in, for me to qualify as a work out the exercise needs to last 20 minutes or travel a distance of a mile. Here is my typical day in my program. When I wake up in the morning the first place I go is into the hot tub for 10 minutes. This just warms up my muscles, this does not constitute a work out. From the hot tub, I go into the pool, I generally swim 10 breaststroke laps to get loosened up. Then I walk 40 lengths of the pool, from there I will alternate days from upper body and lower body workouts. The upper body workout consists of three sets of 100 water push-ups, three sets of 25 seated weighted ball L raises, three sets of 50 sitting rows with water dumbbells, three sets of 50 downward butterflies' then three sets of 50 horizontal butterflies'. I walk 20 lengths of the pool between sets so when I am finished I will have done 100 lengths of the pool walking then I finish it off with ten more laps of the breast stroke as a warm down. That constitutes on work out, next I would either walk the complex perimeter two to three times each lap is one mile, that would constitute a work out, then I head home for a smoothie to get my energy back up, resting in the meantime then it is off to the fitness center where I would do a mile on the treadmill, six minutes on the rowing machine and three miles on the bike, that would-be workout number three. The fourth workout is generally after dinner and would consist of either 20 laps of walking in the pool or a lap around the complex. My activity on the Garmin would dictate what I did after dinner if I was short on steps I would hit the pool, if the temperature was too hot I would hit the pool. It was my choice.

Natural or Nothing? This is a huge debate, depends on who you talk to or what day of the week it is. Remember we live in the land of free enterprise. I remember back in the day way back when we wouldn't touch granola because it wasn't done yet. Back then it looked like ingredients you would use for cookies. Now they slap the word organic on it and double the price for virtually the same product as the one next to it. Ok before I get sued again, if it says organic, most of the time it is. Hopefully that satisfies the masses. But seriously, there is a huge difference between a processed product and a naturally grown product. Like I said earlier in the book, pretty much all food starts out in a natural state, then depending on how long it needs to take from the time it leaves the plant till the time it hits your plate depends on how many preservatives need to be used to achieve that. Remember the number one rule for any manufacturer is to not kill its clients. So, as I drive thru the great state of Nebraska right now. I am surrounded by corn fields as far as the eye can see. It makes me wonder where will all this corn go? You know the farmers just didn't put it in the ground and tend to it all summer just to see it go to waste. Now without getting into the boring details on how many products are made with corn. When you think about it we are probably talking millions of acres of corn are grown each year in the United States. Pretty much all of it is grown in the ground, wouldn't that still make it a natural product? According to the FDA not so much, it is pretty much based on what type of fertilizer is used during the growing stage and what chemicals are used on it during and after it is harvested. I feel a huge B.S. coming. Have we gotten so out touch with reality that we are breaking down food into regular, organic, and beyond. We live in the fattest time in our history, yet we feel the need to spend more money to buy organic menu items for dinner, while we stuff processed menu items down your pie hole off the burger world drive thru at lunch. That is why I am a firm believer that natural is always better than processed. If your kids want more fruits and vegetables give them more. In my 51 years on this planet I have never seen a person die from eating too many fruits or vegetables. Wait but what about the natural sugar found in fruit? Don't worry the diet soda you are slurping down with your pineapple should neutralize it hahahahahahah. There is a HUGE difference between the sugar found in fruit and putting two heaping spoonsful of sugar on your naturally sweetened cereal in the morning. Yes, sugar is sugar, Right! Not in my book, again I am not a doctor, dietician, or a scientist, I am just a fat guy that has chased a dream for the past 40 years or so to live in a healthy body. So, long story short, natural, organic or processed. Read the label, know what you're putting in your body and for God sake parents please know what you are putting in your kid's body. I know for me natural is the direction I am heading. Here is an ah ha tip, I can share with you, if you are not sure which product is organic, gluten free or special. It's the one that is double or so the price of the regular brand. Read both packages, they probably have the same ingredients in them, minus how they achieved that outcome. My wife brought up a great point about the pricing. If they are using less chemicals on the products, why are we paying more money for them than the ones that are using the chemicals? Trust me if the price was the same I would choose the one without the chemicals, but it seems a little opportunistic to prey on healthy people to have to make that choice. Just my opinion. So, I just had an ah ha moment. We just left the hotel that we stayed last night less than an hour ago, I have to plug the Best Western in Kearney, Nebraska it was the nicest Best Western I have ever stayed at. My sister, brother in law and I ate at their continental breakfast before hitting the road. They had a very nice selection of good food, we all seemed to get our fill. So, an hour into our journey back to Michigan my sister asks my brother in law for a breakfast bar. My first reaction is WTF, Right!! But being the caring nurturing brother I am asked politely, hey fat ass why you eating again. Lol She replied on cue Bite Me!! Then we had a normal conversation about why she was eating again. She said she was a bit of an eater when she is bored. Plus, she had a craving for a little chocolate. A little chocolate is not a bad thing if it ties you over till your next big meal. That just adds fuel to my theory to reboot your system. Listen to your body, eat when it is hungry not when you think it needs to eat, there is a huge difference. Let it tell you then feed it, be prepared at all times with a little something something of the healthy variety so if you are not in a situation that you can stop for a meal, at least you can satisfy your hunger. Another good tip is to keep a bottle water with you, sometimes hunger signals sent by your stomach doesn't always mean you're hungry it could mean you're thirsty. Just because your mouth isn't dry or even your throat, your stomach is the organ that processes the water and ships it where it needs to go. Give it water first if the hunger persists then feed it.

The power of suggestion or NOT!!! How many times have I mentioned that you cannot influence a person into doing something they don't want to? Yes, you can threaten them to do it, but the chances of them having the results you want them to achieve probably won't be the same. You can drop subtle hints for them and based on their intelligence level, they may or may not get it. Men how come women have no problem telling us when we are getting fat? But if we don't lie to them that the dress they have chosen to wear for dinner makes their butt look big? WTF I am staying out of that conversation, remember I'm not Dr. Phil. I have noticed that I have cut my television time down to minutes a day now. I could probably go without it completely and not miss it very much. I know I eat a lot less when I don't have awesome looking food paraded in front of me at 60 inches in 4k definition. The only thing missing is the smell of the pepperoni or the sizzle of the steak. Just wait smellovision is not too far away. Then what in the hell are fat people going to do to avoid that. Put down the remote and hit the streets. I know, I'm tired I have been on my feet all day... Wait hear that it's the wambalance!! Outside your door. No one said it was going to be easy. This is your body talking!! Hey fat ass, remember me I'm the one that carried you around all day at work that helped you earn the money that paid for that double Whopper with cheese extra-large value meal you shoved down your pie hole. Now you think you are going to crash on the couch for a couple hours and watch finely tuned athletic machines chase the pig skin around before you drag me off to bed for a couple hours of sleep, then wash and repeat. Bull Shit!!! That is a recipe for disaster, watching sports on tv is almost as bad as watching them at the stadium. At least on tv, you don't have to smell them as you walk by the tailgating or the food vendors. It seems though every commercial during the game makes reference to food or drink can I get an Amen!! Turn off the TV!! Put down the remote, go for a walk worst case scenario, here's one for you go to bed. Like your body couldn't use a couple more hours of sleep. Trust me a rested body will give you a lot more of what you want then a broken down tired one. Just saying!

Here is an ah ha moment that would Segway here nicely from our power of suggestion into Treasure hunting 2.0. so, I said before you never know what you will find treasure hunting. I told you about the $400 juicer I picked up at a garage sale, but I'm not sure if I told you the rest of the story. So, this fit in perfectly to the week I was having talking about juicing. So, I walk into this sale and it was at the end of the day, the ladies just ordered take out and were starting to wind down the sale. When I noticed a

Kitchen aid box kinda sitting under a table, pretty packed up. I asked the lady what she wanted for the Kitchenaid and she informed me that it was a juicer that I am assuming her current husband God rest his soul. Lol Because she was a bigger lady, had bought for her on their anniversary. He came home gave it to her and said here is a hint... Wait for it, wait for it, even I called bull shit on that one. I was afraid even to ask the price of it, much less say anything as stupid as what she did to him. Yes, she informed him that he wasted his money and she would never under any circumstances EVER use it, then she proceeded to ask him how much he spent, so she could take that amount of his money and go buy something she actually wanted. I said you go girl, gave her the $20.00 and was on my way. Take away from this one is gentlemen, unless you are flawless and in top physically fit. Never I repeat never give your lady a weight loss related item for any reason if you want to keep them as your lady. Love them unconditionally and support them all the days of their lives but unless you're bat shit crazy keep away from the weight loss products.

Treasure hunting 2.0 I talk a lot about our Saturday Treasure hunting excursions. In laymen's terms garage sailing. The 2.0 part was modern technology added. When I was, younger I would garage sale with my mom, she was a master at sailing. We would just drive around looking for garage sale signs, one time we were driving behind this one car and my mom said I think this car looks like a sailor, so she followed it all the way to a garage sale and the car drove past the sale. I just shook my head and tipped my hat to the master. Back on track, so in 2016 my sister has an app on her phone that tells you all of the sales within a predetermined range. We would look up the address then have OnStar give us turn by turn directions to our destination. My mother would be proud! Now to the point, you never know what you will find at any given sale. As we travel back to Michigan in a loaded down SUV, I am a testament to that theory. Considering I had to leave some of my treasures back in Vegas because they wouldn't fit in our vehicle. On the kitchen equipment front I scored a $400 Breville Juicer, an emulsifier a Cuisinart food processor. I found great fitness items of which I think my $5.00 weight vest was my most beneficial. I found several hand weights and gadgets that made my workouts more exciting and not so boring. I got a lot of cool souvenirs for the family, they should be pleased, Garage sales are a great resource for fitness equipment, remember everyone has to have the latest and greatest of everything usually the equipment you find at a sale has little or no use on it. On a side note, I would go to the pool extra early on Saturdays to get my workout done, so I would be ready at 7am to head for the sales. I never skipped a workout to go sailing.

Hey Big sexy: Just a side note, this is my nickname and it has been that for years. When you deal with a lot of kids, it's easier to have a nickname then your actual name. I guess it's better than being called fat ass all the time. For me Big Sexy wasn't a bad nickname but my wife and youngest daughter hated when people called me that. Just for the record, fat people would rather be called by their given name then all the adjectives people come up with. Big guy, tubby, jumbo, lard ass, wide load and the list goes on and on and on. If you can't remember their first name sir or ma'am would be sufficient. You would be calling them that out of respect and not out of a weight reference. Just a thought. I believe these two young men gave me the nickname Big Sexy.

24 hours 365 days a year. That is the amount of time I consider I can fit my workouts into one year. Yes, we all have things we have to do other than workout, but these are still the hours available throughout the day, week, month, and year that you can still do your workout if you want to. Leaving the comforts of Resort Villas was very difficult, when you have full access to a gated community with a heated pool and state of the art fitness center that was open 24 hours a day. there were less opportunities for excuses and more opportunities to get a workout done. Coming back to Michigan will increase the excuses on why not to so I will have to fight the urges to give into the excuses and get the work done. I know for the fact that the workout facility I plan to use is only open 5am – 9pm m-f and 6-6 sat. 12-6 on Sundays. So, this will mean I will have to adapt to more of a land workout. Another thing I will have to factor in will be the weather. Considering the three or so months I spent in Vegas the average temperature was over 90 degrees and we only had one day where it rained during the day. Michigan on the other hand has already slipped into the fall, so I would think the temps will average the high 60's until the snow starts flying. Now the big test for me, is hunting season. I'm an avid hunter and my season starts October 1st, through January 1st. no I don't hunt every day, and even when I do, I can walk during the middle of the day, with orange on of course. Really don't want some drunk ass hunter to take a potshot at this fat guy, even though he probably could eat good all winter on what's on my bones lol

Going through the motions: You ever feel like you're going through life on autopilot? I know I did, to me that coincides with living in other people's worlds. It is so easy to get caught up in the grind of the everyday. Now add in a spouse and a couple of kids and your day just went from crazy to off the chain. Did I miss the orientation day when they handed out the life is going to be hard memo? We created the organized chaos we call our lives. We can continue to twist in the wind or we can put our big kid panties on and take the bull by the horns and kick some ass! Did I get enough metaphors in there for you? If I learned even one thing from Chef Claude, it would have to be in preparation for the week is key. Giving yourself a game plan will uncomplicated if nothing else that burning question "what's for dinner." Knowing that will help you shop and prep your meals for the week and just because you make a menu for the week doesn't mean that you can't be flexible with it. The only advice I can give with being flexible with your menu, is take everyone into consideration when preparing it, changing it everyday defeats the reason to have one in the first place. This tool is designed to make things easier for you not make it harder. There are a ton of free sites on the internet with menu options that even include shopping lists. The tools are out there; you just have to go get them. Yes, it's gonna be so time consuming!!! You have the rest of your life to take care of you, make the choice how long you want to do it. For me the longer I can take care of me the happier I get!!!

Unanswered prayers. I might need to apologize in advance for this rant, I can't remember if I put it in at the beginning of the book or not, that is the problem with getting older, having a brain injury and being fat, my CRS sometimes gets the best of me. This rant is worth repeating if it sounds familiar to you again I am sorry. If you are religious or not is irrelevant, we are always asked to say a prayer for someone or something every day. I find it most hypocritical, when politician even as powerful as the president says God bless America at the end of every speech. Yet every chance they get they are looking to remove God from everything we come in contact with so we are not offended by his name. Seriously!!! I am more offended by the groups trying to remove him from everything then God being only targeted when we need him. Okay back to my original rant. Sometimes we get a chance to stop and reflect on how we got to the place we are in life. I mentioned before that everyone has a story and some of the pages in our story are not always filled with sunshine and unicorns, right? Sometimes just the fact that we lived through those days are not special enough for us to feel good. For me I call these my dark side days. The fact that any of us are alive today is a blessing, I know we are not supposed to question why things happen the way they do, and that bad things happen to good people. I get that. Sometimes we think, hey God, I have enough shit on my plate right now, can you give it a break for a bit. That doesn't always help matters either though. It's at those times that we start questioning our very existence and then the what if's start lurking around every thought we take and inevitably that question pops into your head, what if I was dead? Would it really be such a bad thing? No more worries (for me) no more cares (for me) no more pain (for me) who really cares (for me). And this is where God's plan takes over. If you are still here reading this book and I am still here writing it, then at least my prayer was unanswered. I know that I prayed on more than one occasion that God would take me from this world. That he would spare me the worries, stress, and pain, I was experiencing and when he didn't at first I figured he was just busy and he would get to it when he had a chance. It took nearly two and a half years before my body decided to take this journey to get healthy. It wasn't until June 28th, 2016 that my prayers to get healthy started to happen in my life. Now nearly four months later, they are continuing and going strong. There is no scientific or medical reason why I have been able to do what I am doing and yes, I have had some people tell me it is the power of the mind, but again remember I had a brain tumor that started all this problem for me in the first place. Since this is my story, I am going with, unanswered prayers and the prayers that were answered. The thing we must all remember when faced with the decision to take your own life, is yes it may solve your problems. But what about the problems you leave behind for others to clean up? Is it fair to them? There are places you can call, people you can talk to. There is always someone who has it worse than you do. Don't give up, you have so much to offer the world and sometimes you don't even know what you still have to accomplish and you never will if you are not still around to accomplish them. Just saying.

Happily, ever after. What if happily ever after doesn't exist? Does it mean that we can't live as happy as we want too? I don't mean you can't have the fairy tale ending if it means that much to you. I'm just saying, why do we put so much undue stress on ourselves to have something so make believe. Again, I think this stems from our childhood, where prince charming is supposed to come sweep you off your feet on his white horse and you are supposed to ride off to happily ever after land, right? Then as we get older our sights change and get a little more realistic. At least for guys they do. In high school, we are looking to date the head cheerleader or at least make out with her or say that we did. Am I close? I think by the time we graduated, that ship has sailed on most of us. Not for the women though, they still want that fairytale wedding before her life is complete. Again, it's a lot of undue pressure, stress, and money for one day in my opinion. I know it is supposed to be the biggest day of our lives? But shouldn't we treat every day as the biggest day of our lives? Remember we are not guaranteed any more tomorrows. Live in the now and cherish every day like it's the last one you will ever have. That way if it is, you will not go out of this lifetime without any regrets. Just saying

Y'all come back now ya hear. Wow, I just came back from dinner at the fat man's mothership. Now I am not judging and I am not looking to too put anyone down. Remember, just because I have lost 100 lbs. I am still very fat at just under 300 lbs. So, I qualify to be a member of this crowd. Tonight, my wife went out to dinner at Logan's Steakhouse in Muskegon, MI. This has only been the second time since I have been back to Michigan that I have eaten out. The first time was my walk to the diner from deer camp and now this adventure. I never really noticed the size of the people that frequent these types of restaurants. Like I said, they were my size of people. The first thing I thought when we were seated and my eyes adjusted to the dimly lit dining area, I feared for any slow-moving skinny people that might not move quick enough to avoid an errant knife and fork. Lol They were outnumbered and outgunned. The thing was, the customers didn't care very much about the size difference, or the amount of food that they ordered. Let's just say, there wasn't a shortage of cow leaving the building. I almost felt embarrassed ordering a salad for dinner at a steakhouse. I could almost hear the snickers from the peanut gallery. "look at that poser, ordering a salad." But that was it, a salad with chicken, that's all I could come up with. Yes, I could have had anything on the menu, my wife even tried her best to talk me out of ordering it, but I was determined to stay the course and stay the course I did. See, I am trying to be normal, and live a normal life since starting this journey. I told her I would go out to eat with her anytime she wanted as long as I got to order what I wanted, no questions asked. For the most part she has been supportive. Tonight, she gave me crap, but she ordered a salad also, so who was the Jedi knight tonight. Lol to be honest with you the salad was good and filling, the chicken had a nice spice to it and I had it with vinegar and oil, so it wasn't bad for me either. I really wasn't disappointed in my choice tonight. I honestly think chain steakhouses are too pricey on their steaks. I prefer to eat steak at home, because I can get a better cut of steak, for the fraction of the cost. The hardest thing about the entire dinner service, was when they brought out the hot buttered sweet, dinner rolls and of course the waitress sat them down in front of me. That was a killer, I quickly moved them to my wife's side of the table. I actually at one point asked my wife if she was done with them, so I could have the waitress remove that temptation. As we finished our meal and paid the bill, my wife reminded me about the reason we were out there in the first place. To return an item to the mall, yippee the mall. I informed her that I was going to get an ice cream when we got there, to which she replied "I will believe it when I see it". I was prepared and even looking forward to it. I figured I had earned it, I worked out today and have eaten good for almost four months. Time to reward myself, right? So, we get to the mall, this is my wives mothership. She loves to shop, so I follow her lead and let her go first. I didn't want to look too eager if I made a beeline to the ice cream shop. Low and behold, she knows how OCD I can get if I am made to wait, so she headed their first. Just my luck we get to the DQ, and there is a line from hell, the other fat people from dinner must have heard me and beat me to the finish line. She muttered those famous last words, "do you want to wait or come back?" I reluctantly said let come back later, so we beamed back aboard the shopping craft, and went along our merry way. So about two hours and three or four or five stores later, but who's counting. My wife was finished and we headed back towards the ice cream shop. Much to her surprise, I made a right at the store where we came in at. She quickly reminded me about the ice cream, I told her I was so over it now and I was all good. I could see by her expression she was shocked that I would give up that easily on ice cream. But I don't allow anything to have control over me anymore, especially not an empty calorie food item. So maybe this will help her realize how committed I am to getting healthy. I know my body appreciated it, I'm sure it figured I would want to work out extra hard tomorrow if I cheated on it today and it would be right. Lol

If tomorrow never comes? Do you see a pattern here? Other than the fact Garth Brooks is one of my favorite singers, his songs speak to me on a higher level. They make me sit back and wonder, what if? Without going dark again, how many times or how often do you think to yourself, what if tomorrow never comes? I guess on a selfish sadistic way; I wouldn't have to worry about working out tomorrow then. But seriously, have you accomplished everything you wanted to in your lifetime? Are you ready for it to be over? Are you ready for someone else to tell you it is over? Then why do we do the things we do to shorten our life expectancy? I know it's a delicate balance between risk and reward. Remember life isn't worth living, unless you are living your life? So, we can't live in a bubble hoping that nothing bad happens to us, right? But if we shovel loads of toxic crap down our throats while we are in that bubble are we still as safe as we think we are? If it is true that weight loss is 80% nutrition and 20% exercise is that too much to ask us to focus on daily? I can honestly say no or hell to the no!! If that works better for you. I am not asking you to stop eating anything, nor am I saying you need to spend every waking hour sweating your ass off in a gym. All I am asking; is you make the choice to take your own journey to a healthier you. Whatever that looks like on you. That is all I can hope for you, is that maybe reading this book will spark something in you, to motivate you to choose life and live it to its fullest. The second hope I have for you, is that you get right with the loved ones in your life. This is from my dark side, statistics have proven that fat people live shorter lives and without pointing fingers, we pretty much did this to ourselves. We really don't have the right to hold our loved ones responsible for our weight issue. Tell them that you love them, every chance you get. Skinny people die all the time too. Death does not discriminate either, sometimes it may feel like he picks on us a little more. Probably because we have such a big target on our backs. Just saying

Sex? That's a stupid question. This may be breaking "guy code" but for the importance sex plays as a motivational tool for men. It is well worth breaking the code. I mentioned early that men are a simple creature, yes, we are not all the same and yes there are liars among us too. But basically, for most of my species, we could live off the four major food groups. Food, beer, sex, and sports. Not always in that order, but close. I can't speak for all men, but for some of us our lives would be complete if we were eating pizza, drinking beer while having sex during a commercial during the super bowl. Jackpot!!! No that is not romantic, I didn't say anything about making love, I said sex. There is a difference. So, you may be getting ready to scream bull shit, on so many levels right now. I hear you, where would you like me to start? Let's start with the obvious, how men and women view sex. There is no denying that, women are looking to make a connection while making love, most men are just so surprised it is happening, we are just going with it. I can't speak for all women, I can't speak for any of them, since I am not one nor have I ever been one. But considering I have been married to one for almost thirty years now. I was raised with six sisters and I have 51 years of experience dealing with women, I feel a bit qualified. In my experience sex and the use of sex either as a positive or negative motivation tool sucks!!! No pun intended. They had this question on Family Feud a while back, what would a man do for sex? The answers didn't surprise me any, lie, pay, beg, kill and the number one answer was die for it. Lol Now I have never heard that question asked about what women would do for it. I wouldn't think the answers would not be anywhere as funny or extreme as their male counterparts were. I told you earlier women are smarter than men, so I got that out of the way early. It is for that reason; I caution you now. When sex is used against most men, two things generally happen okay maybe three things. One, you piss us off and kill whatever motivation we have to want to please you or us for that matter. Two, you send us out into the world looking for an alternative. Remember Trixie, she isn't still in business because she like doing it so much, it's because she has so many customers and the money is good. Or three we take matters into our own hands and I will leave it at that. Now without being crude, this statement is as true today as it was in my teens when I was first told it, again I apologize in advance, "women have half the money and all the pussy" Another one of God's cruel jokes. No, that's not always the case with the money part, but the second half of the equation, is a definite. Now reverting to my Spiderman days. With that power, comes responsibility! Yes, you have the ability to control men with sex or lack of it. The equalizer to your control is every woman has one. Just saying. Better hope you have a female judge for your divorce proceedings, because you won't get the sympathy vote from a male judge when sex or lack of it rears its ugly head in his court room. Pun intended. As for what does this have to do with weight loss? Everything, Sex is one of the things we would die for. Love us for who we are and what we are. Deep down under all that skin is the person you fell in love with. For whatever reason, life happened and we became this. With your love and support we will become that person again, don't give up on us. Remember those words we said, for better or worse, richer, or poorer, in sickness and health? Obesity is a sickness, it may be bad now, but there is a great chance it will get better and I am going to start that journey TODAY!!

Stop Thinking!! Why we are on the subject, stop thinking!! Men live for sex. It is one of our primal needs. Ask 100 men these questions and you got it 99 will say don't care and you guessed it one liar. I have a headache, don't care. I need to shower, don't care. Aunt flow is here, don't care. My butt is big, don't care. The neighbors are watching, tell them to go home!! Lol okay the last one was a little creepy but it doesn't matter to a man, okay not all men. Another misconception is lingerie, over rated. Just another obstacle we need to chew through to get to the good stuff. Edible under pants were made with fat guys in mind. But again, other than that missed midnight snack, why add calories to an already satisfying process. By over thinking we complicate everything. Take weight loss for instance. With a million products, diets, programs, gimmicks, and guru's how do you know which one is best? You don't, we complicate it so much to the point of overload or until we say screw it and decide it is too complicated and don't do it at all. How about trying these three little tips to help you get healthy? One, listen to your body! It's that big fleshy thing that keeps all the shit inside you, that you need to exist. You know the one we stopped listening to years ago, because life happened and we started flying solo. Two, stop putting toxic shit down your throat. Read the labels, that's what they are there for, if it doesn't have a label, there is probably a good reason for it. Figure out what your body needs and give it to it. It will tell you if it likes it or not. And three, get moving, sitting on the couch watching some finely tuned athletic specimens chase the pigskin around for hours, doesn't count as physical activity for you. Get out walk, workout, swim do whatever activity that you can do to get your heart rate up and yes, sex does and is proven to be a weight loss tool. Amen, just saying. Now that I think about it, I could list a ton more things that would help you on your journey, but like I just got through saying use the KISS method, Keep It Simple Stupid. Don't overthink it, don't over estimate it and don't overdo it. Everything in moderation!! A little bit of something other than arsenic is better than a whole lot of something that will kill you slower. YOU are the only thing your body needs right now. You to take control over you and do what's best for you. But fat guy, there are other people I need to take care of. You are so right, but who's going to take care of them when there is no you around to do it?

Got sick? Sickness is a great way to derail us off our journey. I have been fortunate enough. Other than the pulled muscle in my back, to stay relatively healthy so far. I know I my ass still hasn't rebounded yet from that spinning class I took a couple of weeks ago, Lol I know inevitably it will happen, sickness is everywhere, germs are like calories, anytime you are around a lot of people you still run the risk of being infected. You would think if my main exposure to people is at the gym, my chances of getting sick would be lower, since don't only healthy people workout? Seriously? This is another misconception, show me any healthy gym member and I am sure there is a picture somewhere of their former self that doesn't resemble the person they are today. Most of them started out frail, misguided gym rats, from a previous life and through the cocoon process blossomed into the fine specimen you see today. Seriously? No, but it sounded better than saying through hard work and being committed to their journey, they have become what they are today. Not as glamorous but effective just the same. I don't know if the vitamins and the E-mergenC is what has kept me healthy so far, it could be the food I have chosen to put into my body or the exercise I am doing. Or a combination of all of it, not sure. But if it keeps me out of the doctor's office and healthy, I'm not going to question it!! I had a football coach once, that was a hard ass. He would always tell us, "he got sick once, he didn't like it much, so he never got sick again." I knew him for a long time and as long as I knew him he never missed a day of football or work. He died of brain cancer, when he was in his 80's. Maybe he stored all that sickness for all those years up in his head, until one day it killed him. The power of suggestion. The brain is a powerful tool, when used to do good. Just Saying

Can't the worst four letter word in our vocabulary. I can't stand when every word out of a
fat person's mouth is CAN'T. hahahahahah If fat people said I can't eat another bite before they started eating how great would that be? So now that I have used the word can't four times in the first four sentences, let me expand on it. Being an old time coach the word I hated the most besides lost is can't. there really isn't anything you can't do if you put your mind to it. Think about it, I just drove from Michigan to Vegas and back in five days. Back in the day it would have taken the early settlers months to go coast

to coast. Sure, I could have flown there in 5 hours but it was so much more enjoyable in the car, said no grown ass man EVER!! Take and scenario that you would say can't to and think about it, I bet you could figure out how to change the outcome to did or can. For example, if I told you to pick up this car with everything inside it. At first you would think the fat guy is off his meds, right? If you tried to pick it up by yourself, I would think you were off your meds. Now expand your brain, a tow truck could pick this truck up, a forklift could a floor jack could, so it's not impossible right, driving through the mountains was an amazing experience. I'm sure at one time in our history someone has said we can't get to the other side of these mountains, but we just did in a matter of hours. 99.9% of the time it's not that we couldn't it's that we didn't do it right. You must be able to adapt to your environment, overcome the obstacles that are in your way and have that never say never and whatever it takes attitude it takes to get the job done. You are dealing with your very existence here; the choice is life or death for most of us. Choose life and don't take no for an answer. Many people think fuck is the worst word in the English language, I would challenge you that Can't is way worse.

Cooked or Raw? Depends on what it is, to stay out trouble with the legal team, I'm going to have to revert back to the standard response please make sure you cook raw meats to the proper and safe cooking temperatures before consuming them. Remember rule number 1 no one wants to die for the food they eat. On the flip side, clean raw vegetables stay in their most nutritious state un cooked. The longer you cook them the more taste and nutrition you cook out of them. Chef Claude turned me onto a great tasting healthy menu choice before I left. Did you know cabbage and celery are the two vegetables that eaten raw burn more calories than you consume eating them. So, I was all over this white on rice. It is very simple to make and yes before you ask the olive oil does add calories but again if I can eat a plate of this for under 100 calories is that a bad thing. Take one medium green cabbage wash it, core it and chop it. I put it in my $14.00 food processor with the shredder attachment on, shred the entire head, put the entire head of shredded cabbage into a Ziploc bag, drizzle a half cup of olive oil into the bag and put one tablespoon of crushed black pepper in the bag and shake it up and lay it in the refrigerator. The ingredients will marry together, I would continue to shake the bag occasionally, but that's it, eat it whenever you want, I added some balsamic vinegar to mine before I ate it, but I found it to be delicious

Happy Hours: There is one thing I learned about the Villas, the ladies liked their happy hours. All I can say is if drinking is bad for you, sign me up. A couple of prime examples of the positive effects of alcohol was Renee, she was one of my skinny friends I threatened to eat her all the time. Our standard joke was inside every fat person was a skinny person because we ate them so we didn't have to hear how fat they thought they were. lol She was the size four that bought a dress for her son's wedding a couple sizes too small and worked her ass off literally to fit into a size 0 dress. Renee is in her 60's but you would never know it, as her new granddaughter put it so eloquently, she is hot!! Renee's drink of choice is a NorCal. Made with tequila, club soda and lime. I was too much of a sissy, to try that one. Renee never stops, she is always on the go, she is an incredible woman. Another one of my drinking buddies was Ms. Betty, she loves wine. Ms. Betty is around 80. She too never stops. She does water aerobics, yoga, and Pilates. She loves life, she tells me that I'm her inspiration but I tell her all the time that she is mine, remember up until about three months ago, I didn't expect to make it to see the new year. Now I am hoping to live the same life as they have. Claude's mother drinks a glass of wine a day and lives on her own in France at age 89 so there is scientific proof that alcohol in moderation is not a bad thing. I guess it's time to fess up on the drinking buddy comment, I had a total of six Corona's and one rum and pineapple juice on my journey, so this chapter was about the effects of alcohol on other people. I just didn't want to set myself up for them to call B.S. on me because I'm such a cheap date. Lol

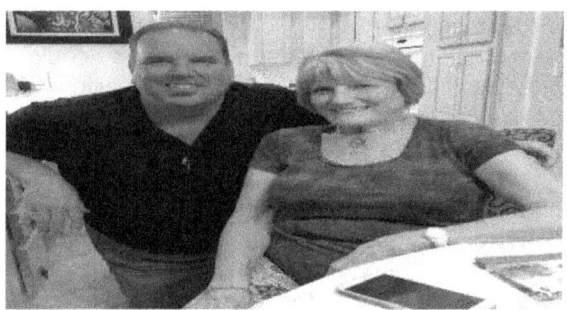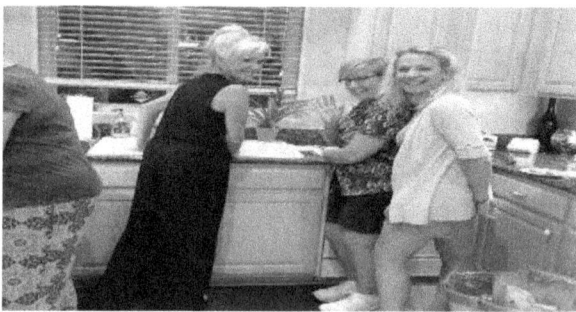

Back to life, back to reality: Well I am back to Michigan and pretty much my biggest fears became reality. It is Thursday afternoon on day 87. I have been able to work out a total of five hours the entire week so far. Life came back with a vengeance, between trying to fix a broken riding mower so I could cut the jungle that used to be my lawn. Starting physical therapy again, having a MRI done this morning. Covering my buddy's shop this afternoon and a couple of meetings this week so far, it has been pretty much a cluster to say the least. On a positive note my weight loss has continued even though I haven't been able to work out that much. I stepped on the scale yesterday morning at the Tamarac where I do my workouts now and I weighed 312 lbs. So, I lost another three pounds through all the traveling. That puts me at 88 lbs. total on the journey to date I attribute my continued weight loss on what I am putting in my mouth. I have continued on my current game plan of menu items and portion control. No empty calories, plenty of water and resting my body as needed. Monday morning, I took on the task of weed whipping the yard, I can honestly say I sweat more that day alone then I did in the 79 days I spent in Vegas that had experienced their hottest June & July on record I may add. I considered pausing the weight loss clock as of the Thursday we left Vegas and pick it back up next Monday when I can start working out full time again, but I didn't want to affect the integrity of the journey that I am on to reach my goal in 100 days. I may have to add an asterisk after the 100 days if I don't reach my goal in the allotted time. But we will cross that bridge when we get there. As of right now I have 13 days to lose 12 pounds and that is my focus.

New home sweet home: So now that I have left the confines of Resort Villas, it was time to find a new place to spend countless hours to finish chapter one of this journey. The Tamarack Wellness Center is where I returned to. This is my old stomping ground. I do my therapy there as well, I have already spent about as much time in the pool here over the past three years as I did this past summer at the Resort Villas. I intend to do more land work now since they have an indoor track as well as a fitness center. Another tool that I have added to my workout tool kit is the sauna. They have a very nice wet sauna; I spend 15 minutes in the sauna before I hit the pool and 15 minutes after I get out of the pool before I head into the gym to do my land workout. I have met some interesting people in just the short time I have started working out there again. The facility does a lot of specialized fitness classes. They do an extreme workout class with an instructor named Courtney. Her students push themselves to the extreme every second of that class. I would think that there are on average 16 students in that class, one guy, eight skinny girls and seven larger but ex-jock built girls. I talked to the instructor and asked her if I provided the journals would she encourage her students to participate in my research project. I would like them to journal for one week, their weight loss and everything they eat that week. I will be very interested first on how many will actually take the time to do it, second how many will actually tell the truth about what they are eating. I also asked them to share their weight loss journey and any successes and failures they may have encountered along the way. I will then compile the data they provide me and add it to my next book called "Chapter two, the second 100." I will keep you updated on the progress to that also.

Swimming with the fishes: So, I think I have pretty much come full circle on all the pool time I have logged these past three years or so. In the beginning, I used to get so irritated by people that walked in the pool when I was doing a majority of my working out swimming. It seemed to never fail when you spend as much time as I do in the pool that you have to adjust your workout around others when you share a public pool. So, I adapted and kept on keeping on as they say. But over this past three months or so, I have realized how beneficial walking in the pool has been for me, I wish I would have utilized it much earlier in my workout routine. It's been awhile since I have called B.S. so here it is. Anyone that thinks they are going to lose weight floating in a weightless environment and wiggle your toes and flail your arms and call that swimming BBBB to the SSSSSS!!! Now before I get Michael Phelps, tracking me down looking to kick my fat ass, let me clarify this. Yes, if you spend over eight hours in the pool at a time, and train like you are qualifying for the 2020 Olympics yes there is a benefit there. Again, if you are floating on your back letting the current from the walkers creating that current, 0 calories invested. If there is a silver lining to the "workout" you think you are doing. If it keeps you off the couch and stops you from shoving Cheetos down your pie hole waiting to see if he is the father!! Dun dun dun!! Then I guess that is a positive. But for me, swimming the amount of laps I have swam have gotten me stronger in the muscles that I have used to get me from end to end but not so much when it came to weight loss. Remember though this is your journey, if you feel it is working for you by all means keep on keepin on!!

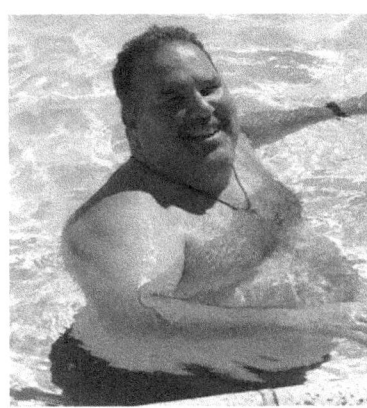 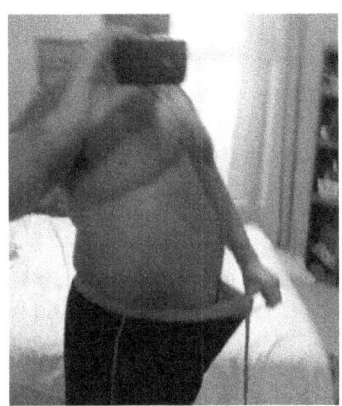 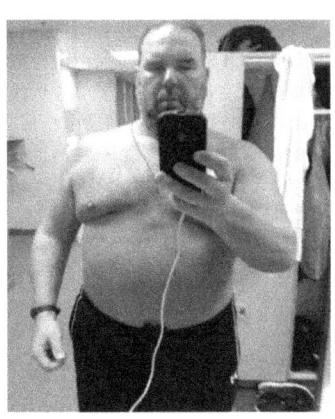

For all that is holy, Look the part: This might be a pet peeve of mine, but since this is my journey, I feel the need to call B.S. on this subject to. So how many of you out there have gone to fat dietician or a fat personal trainer? Why? I know you're gonna say because they had a degree, or they had experience or even you don't know their story. I can totally understand that and as a person I would never want to sit in judgement of another person's life choices. But for me, I find it very difficult to take advice about nutrition or weight loss from someone that needs to practice what they preach. Again, I hear you, I shouldn't judge others without knowing them. But as a fat guy that has been there and done that. It would be very easy for me to say you need to do this and this and this if you want to get healthy. But the reality to that is I'm still fat, why would you take any advice from me, I am just giving you examples of what I did to achieve the results I have I am not a weight loss guru, or anything like that, I am just a fat guy trying to make a difference in a world of fat people that may think that it's too late or not possible for them to lose weight themselves. When it comes to the skinny part to this whole journey. You control where it goes and where it doesn't if you are strong you can go far. If you are weak and allow others to control your journey you will never know how far they will let you go on your journey

Getting steamed!!! So, since being back in the mitten, I have started using a new tool at my fitness center. The wet sauna is my new best friend. First, let me clarify that, this is the closest thing to hell on a rainy day that I want to come to the real hell. I do 15 mins. In the sauna before I hit the pool, then I do 15 mins. More after the pool before I hit the gym. I set the timer on my watch for 15 mins. Exactly. I don't care if there is anyone in there with me or not. I could be in mid-sentence of a deep conversation and my timer go off and I am out the door. It's pretty much a love / hate relationship. I love the affects the steam room has on my body but I hate sitting in the heat, just sweating if that makes sense? We will have to see how it translates into weight loss after I have done it for a week. Other than that, I call a resounding B.S. to all the macho men that have to be the last one to leave the sauna. It's almost an unwritten man code that is you enter the sauna and there is someone else already in there, that you should stay in there until they leave or you look like a sissy. I call B.S. like I said if sweaty pruney guy wants to sit in hell for 15 mins and 2 seconds, more power to you, just don't get in my way as I head for the door or there's going to be a collision. lol

WTF? <u>Where's the food?</u> While I was in Vegas, there was a man from Arizona that lost over 300 lbs. in three years walking to the grocery store every time he was hungry. His doctor told him if he didn't change his lifestyle he wouldn't see his 30's so he went home and threw all the food out he had at his house and every time he was hungry he walked a mile each way in the heat of Arizona for over a year, then he progressed to working out at a gym to lose the additional weight. He had a great story is name is Pat, they called him fat pat, now they call him possible pat. That is awesome.That brings up a great point, when was the last time you cleaned out your pantry, refrigerator, or freezer? If you're anything like me the answer is when I made my last meal. Seriously when? This might be a great place to start your journey and before I have all the hunger activists screaming kill the fat guy!! I don't mean throw away all of your groceries. There are probably several food pantries in your area that would gladly take your donations, even churches welcome donations for food drives. So, for God sake literally, don't waste good food. As a last resort throw it away, you need to rid yourself from the temptations lurking in your kitchen, remember out of sight out of mind! But if all you have to do is open the door or cupboard how difficult is that? I know the first thing I did the morning after I arrived home was to clean out the refrigerator. I cut up and bagged all the fruit and vegetables we bought the night I got home and prepared for the week ahead, chef Claude would have been so proud. Remember that part of the book early on, when I said lose weight without buying a bunch of special or diet food? This isn't the opportunity to purge your storage area of all your old food and buy a bunch of new diet food. That's not the point here. The point is to limit the temptations around you of any unhealthy or empty calorie food choices, if you can go without replacing them with anything then kudos to you. If you need a substitute for the food you are replacing, then you need to do what you need to do. Remember the key here is to build a trust up with your body, your body should realize when you start making healthy food choices that something has changed. Remember everybody is different, if it doesn't figure it out overnight stay persistent, you didn't put the weight on overnight, don't expect it to come off overnight either. Fruit is my go to between meals, almonds, yogurt and vegetables work as well. If I have a real craving for a little extra something something, I will do a smoothie, you can also add cocoa powder to the smoothie if you need a chocolate boost. In a rare crisis moment give yourself what you want in moderation. Again, chocolate in moderation isn't horrible, a whole bag of chocolate not so much. Sorry Remember if you can go without kudos, if you need some encouragement or reward for good work well done then do what you need. This is your journey, your life, live it on your terms. I found that I was on a mission and nobody or nothing was going to stop me from attaining my goals.

Sauna, Sauna, Sauna, Saturday & Sunday. Well, it's not my favorite two days of the week, but I told you earlier I work out seven days a week. The problem comes in that the place I work out at has open family swim, both Saturday and Sunday. So, in order to get in a good workout, I have to be creative. So, this week I started doing 30, 30, 30. Times two. Lol I do 30 minutes in the sauna, then 30 mins in the gym, 30 more minutes in the sauna then 30 more minutes in the gym. Then yes you guessed it 30 more in the sauna and finish up with 30 more in the gym. If you think about it, that is about half the time I spend working out on a daily basis. I was there at 6am today and out the door by 10am. Plus I sweat my ass off literally. That brings me to my next rant. Who ever said this is fun? Working out is not or never fun, unless you are some deranged skinny person stuck in a masochistic Groundhog Day movie. Working out is a lot of things but it's fun said no fat person ever. It's not supposed to be. Working out really is payback for everything you put your body through on a daily basis. It kills me how many people I hear talking at the gym about all the food they consume over the weekend. But these are the same people that bust their ass's all week trying to lose weight I guess so they can afford to eat so much over the weekend. That makes no sense to me, here is a novel idea, how about cut back on your portion size and eat what you want. Or the next time you are thinking hey I think I will slam a double Whopper down my flapper, why not eat a Whopper Jr. instead and save yourself a couple thousand calories? Trust me I have no room to talk,

I was the fat guy behind you in that line, hoping you would hurry up and make up your damn mind. The menu hasn't changed in years, yet some people ask about everything on the menu, yet in the end order the same thing they always get. Here is another tip, why do we torture ourselves by going to places the give endless refills on some food items? Then we feel obligated to order more just because I paid extra for it dammit, I want it all. Again, this is another reason I seldom eat out, I would rather not feel the temptation to overeat, plus I can cook anything pretty much for less than it would cost to eat out. Since I am on a roll, here is another thing I heard today and I had to scream bull shit!! The commercial announcer was talking about some fitness product, that is you purchased it would make you feel like one of the founding fathers, News flash, I don't care what you do, you are still always going to be you. Stop trying to be something you are not. You see the people that start a new workout routine and they have to go out and buy all new workout clothes. Just cause you're all decked out from head to toe with Under Armor gear. It doesn't make you a member of team UA. If anything, it makes you a poser, yes some of the clothes that they make today is beneficial for working out. Moisture wicking, cool fabric, cross training shoes. I get that part, but other than changing your last name ladies when you get married, you are always going to be you. Yes, you should aspire to be the most fabulous you possible, but other than that, keep it real and be yourself, just saying.

Segment two
The Journey Continues
The Second Hundred
Walking Uphill Both Ways!!

As they say onwards and upwards, I completed journey one in 99 days unofficially!! Remember we really didn't have an official start weight. Because I didn't have access to a scale that would weigh my fat ass. We guessed it was 400, all I know I was damn fat and Vegas was damn hot last summer. When I weighed myself at 5:05am Tuesday October 4, 2016 the scale read 300.00 so that's my story and I'm sticking to it. The thing you most need to remember is this is my story, my journey and I call it as I see it. If you didn't read the title of the book it's called "How I Lost 100Lbs. In 100 Days," You might be a little lost when I refer to some of the things I talked about, in segment one but for all you sequel haters out there, me included… I will keep you in the loop as much as possible without sounding redundant or just plain stupid. Lol This is my journey; I hope this book will inspire you to take your own journey to a healthier life. The following is a bunch of rants that document my journey through life as a fat guy. How I ended up where I started, the middle and where I ended this current journey. This book in no way is the end all be all on weight loss. I still am confused on how I was able to go from over 400 lbs. down to 300 lbs. in 100 days. The biggest message I would like to share with everyone is it is not too late to choose life and to decide to get healthy. If a 51-year-old 400 lb. stroke survivor with balance and vision issues can lose weight. I would challenge you to do the same. Good luck and Godspeed on your journey. Now that the paperwork is finished as they say, we can dive into the second journey. This one is going to be a bit different than the first one, for several reasons. First and foremost, because I'm not as fat as I was last time, second because as of right now I am not in Las Vegas starting the journey. I am in Podunk Hesperia, MI. If you have ever had the pleasure of visiting Hesperia, MI you might have either been lost or drunk. Take your pick. No breathalyzers are going on today, now before all the locals come at this fat guy with their pitchforks at the ready. Let me get a head start in my pickem up truck. Seriously though, I have lived in this small farming community close to 20 years and There are some good folks that live here. They are good people as they like to say here in the sticks. I guess if there has to be a third reason, it's because I had to adapt to a life of working on land and by sea. The fitness center as well as the pool. As for me no real big changes health wise, other than missing a quarter of my weight. The effects of the stroke are still in full force. I still have the same balance and vision issues I had last journey. My neck issues continue to pop up on occasion also. I still am considered disabled by the establishment as of now that is. You never know when we will get threatened about social security benefits being cut or they don't like how your review goes, but as of now I am still rich every fourth Wednesday of the month. Lol,I still workout at the Tamerac Wellness Center in Fremont, MI. It is a multi-functional building owned by Spectrum Health. The building is a converted Wal-Mart department store. Now the building houses a rehabilitation center, that is where I go for physical therapy as well as a fitness center and a pool. It also has a walking track that makes it a very good one stop shopping center for a good workout. Like I said the second half of this book is going to be a bit different in a couple ways. Yes, it's still going to have my smart-ass comments as well as the weight loss through the eyes of this fat guy. But I have also put things in motion to collect data from several of the citizens of the Tamerac. Isn't that cute that they label us as citizens, what if we don't want to be civilized? At any moment, what if we are pushed to the limits and have a craving to eat the first skinny person in sight? Is that grounds to have to give up our citizen card? A valid fat guy question I must say, I am just sorry I failed to ask it at registration. Ok back on subject I still have a tendency to get off subject. So yes, I will continue to share my experiences on this second journey, but I will also be adding experiences from members of the fitness community and what has worked and not worked for them in a keeping it real lingo that we should all be able to play along with. Another change I have added to this journey is a daily journal of my fitness and nutrition from day one all the way to 200 lbs. Lost. It might get a little boring to read, the first three days I have averaged eight hours of workout time each day. Remember nothing has changed from my original mission other than I achieved mission one which was to lose 100 lbs. In 100 days. I told you that was just mission one from the beginning, I am still fat and morbidly obese. Even when I hit my next goal of 200 lbs. I will still be in the establishments eyes obese. That won't deter me from getting there though.I have learned a lot about myself over the last 101 days. Yes, I have always been a bit of a smart ass and yes, I have always been very competitive. But I think the thing that sticks out the most to me is when someone challenges me to do something, mostly when they don't think I can do it. Then I find myself getting pretty pissed off and determined to prove them wrong. For example, my senior year of high school, I broke my ankle in P.E proving I was a bad ass volleyball player right, unfortunately for me it was right before basketball season started so I wasn't able to play basketball, but it didn't mean when the captain of the cheerleading squad asked me to join the cheer team because they needed someone to pick up the cheerleaders, I was all over it like white on rice. So, for some macho types out there, I know you might be saying "so you were a cheerleader?" My response to them is hell to the yes!!! Where else can a hormone in tennis shoes have the opportunity to lift up beautiful girls over their heads every Wednesday and Friday night and get into the basketball games for free. That's not it!! Just for playing along we're going to throw in endless hugs just for playing. So, I think that was the best ankle injury I have ever had. Just saying. So, it shouldn't come as much of a surprise to you then, when I am really going to push myself to get to 200 lbs. Lost in 200 days. What's the worst that can happen? I hit 190 in 200 days, is that so bad. I have to set the goal high so I push myself to do my best right. The only limitation I have put on me right now is to continue to do it healthy and listen to my body the whole way. So, without further ado, let me drop this little gem on you. So, you know I am a firm believer that things happen for a reason. We may not always know what God has planned for us, but when we get hints dropped, we need to run with them. So, it just happens that the day I hit my 100 lb. goal the Tamerac, starts a fall into fitness challenge. The contest runs from October 4th- November 15. So, that works out to 43 days. The goal I have set for myself is 50 lbs. Lost by November 15th. Wish me luck, I'm going to need it. I will keep you updated. With the new challenge, come with it new opportunities to start new classes and workouts. So far, I have done five Tabata classes in the pool. Tabata is a combination of water aerobics and a high-powered cardio program. The premise is to keep your heartrate going for the entire 60-minute class doing 10 rounds of different exercises for 30 seconds on and 10 seconds of rest at a time in between exercises. I do my regular pool workout immediately following that class, it's a killer, believe me. I have also added classes to my land workouts. The main class I am doing meets Monday, Wednesday & Fridays from 8am to 9am. It is called energizers, it is a combination between, dance, aerobics, Zumba with dumbbells mixed in. I know I am fat, I know since the stroke I have no rhythm, now sprinkle in balance and vision issues and you have the perfect storm for something funny or bad to happen. Let's just say I made it through the first class with my life intact, any street cred I may have had going into that class was quickly eliminated when the Macarena came on. Without turning this into a racial issue, did I happen to mention I am white too? For my convenience, the room is lined with mirrors. So, I could see how ridiculous I looked at 360 degrees, let's just say it wasn't pretty. But at the end of the class, I was so happy that I challenged myself to stick it out and I will be back again in the morning.

Walking uphill, both ways: That has always been a strange analogy for me, but we have heard it a million times, especially when you talk to someone from the older generation. It usually is linked to the phrase, "when I was a kid, I used to walk to school for miles uphill both ways." In many ways weight loss is an uphill battle both ways, for some of us the fitness part is a battle or it's the nutritional part that we struggle with. It never feels balanced and for a fat guy both sides suck. Remember I'm an equal opportunity fat guy I hate them both. Lol So now that I established that they both suck, now what? I can't believe I am going to suggest this, because I made it clear in the last book that working out is not fun. "Make it fun." I know B.S., exactly I hear you, I guess there are levels of suckiness make it suck less. For me that is why I start out in the sauna and the hot tub every workout, even though the sauna hasn't made it to my Christmas card list yet, I still see the benefit from sitting in it sweating my ass off literally. The hot tub has always been a reward with benefits, so I start my workouts with things that my body enjoys doing, it is less of a fight for me. You want to kill your motivation completely? Start planning your next day's work out expectations and start the day with a 10-mile run, or 100 push ups' and see how quickly your body will yell B.S. I can only tell you my experience so far and going into day 104 I still have plans to go to the gym after church today, so I haven't found the off button yet. As for the nutritional part of the equation? Experimentation, is my best advice. See what you can live without, try to modify the things you CAN'T live without. Notice the word CAN'T bolded. Before you say you CAN'T, try at least three times to see if you really can't. Telling yourself you can't before you ever try because you have convinced yourself that if I do this is going to happen is B.S. I am 51 years old, I have canted myself plenty of times in my lifetime, without even trying it in the first place and I regret never trying many things earlier in life than now. Example, yesterday I was craving pizza, who was ever said that fat people? Can I get an amen? This has always been one of my guilty pleasures, in essence pizza in general is not a bad product for you. Yes, the cheese can be a bit much, depending on how much you use, what blend it is how much pepperoni is used that the grease pools on the top of it, you know the basics. The toppings can be all natural and the sauce is tomato based. The two killers on pizza in my opinion is the crust and the fact that most of us are not content with eating a couple pieces. For some reason pizza is a menu item that we have to continue to eat until it is gone. A good pizza, is great for dinner, a midnight snack, breakfast, and lunch, consecutively if the supply holds out. Am I lying? So yesterday I was craving it so I tried a new recipe. Eggplant based pizza, now before I get all the Guido's of the world rolling up on me, wanting me to swim with the fishes. I never said this was going to replace pizza to the masses. This was me experimenting with a craving. So, when I was at the farmer's market last week, I found a couple of huge eggplants, probably the biggest ones I have ever seen. They had to be at least seven inches in diameter and 13 inches long. I sliced them into ½ inch sections round and flash froze them and put them in the deep freeze. Last night I pulled a couple out, microwaved them a couple of minutes to soften them up. Rubbed them with olive oil and topped them like I would a regular pizza. (Down Guido) baked them at 400 degrees for 15 mins until the cheese was browned and ate it with a fork and knife. No I couldn't eat it like a slice of pizza, no it didn't taste exactly like pizza, did it satisfy my craving for pizza? You bet it did, No I don't know how many calories or fat grams were in it. I know that I only ate the two slices that I cooked though, no midnight snack, no breakfast or lunch today from the left overs. Will I do it again, most definitely!! "Not if we have anything to say about it" Says every Guido everywhere!!! Lol Oh ya and then my wife and I went on a three-mile walk. Tell me the last time you have eaten pizza for dinner and wanted to do anything after dinner other than unbutton your pants? The moral of the story is don't ever say Can't without trying it first and don't knock it till you try it!!

You are never too old to learn new tricks: I know we hear this all the time and we can do as much or as little or as lot as you want to do. Just be prepared to get as little or as lot back in return for what you are willing to put into it. Challenge yourself to do when you or someone tells you that you CAN'T. I heard something from one of the old-timers at the gym the other day that stuck with me. "Will power is a muscle, you need to exercise it, to make it stronger." I don't know about you but that sounds like challenge to me? Since then whenever I get into that rationalizing argument with myself, you know the one daily. You know the one that sounds like the Clash song "Should I stay or should I go?" instead I change the lyrics to "Should I eat or will I blow it?" Ya, that feeling. I decided every time I get the urge to eat more, or choose something I shouldn't eat, to flex my "Will Power" muscle and stay on the path to skinny and narrow. Remember I am still on coming off my path of the fat & scary. I kind of like this new path better. Another new trick is get your stuff already the night before you head to the gym. I am fortunate the gym I work out at offers a locker and laundry service, for a fee of course. Nevertheless, this has been an argument of mine with my wife since the beginning of my membership here. The $20.00 a month I pay for this service is well worth it to me to have my workout clothes washed and hanging in my locker every day when I arrive at the gym. Then to worry about doing it myself on a daily basis. To break it down into a cheap fat guys rational. I work out almost 30 times a month at least. That is like .67 a day, it would cost me more in detergent and electricity to do that myself. Yes, I could see her point if I used it once a week, but thank God I am fortunate enough to make it financially worth it. As for setting out my clothes the night before, I know it sounds childish. But I know my wife appreciates me not rummaging through my drawers and the closet at four am looking for my crap. Remember eliminate the obstacles in your workout life to maximize your losing potential. I just had an ah ha moment. I just realized I have spent most of my life trying to be a winner, maybe this is part of the reason my body fights being a loser? The competitor in my HATES yes, I used that word again hates to ever lose, I guess even when losing is a good thing. I guess I will have to change losing weight to getting healthy and see how that feels instead. I mentioned earlier that I asked a group of people at the gym to journal their weight loss experience for me and why and how they have decided to do what they are doing to try to get fit. I asked them to write down their weekly nutrition and fitness activities as well as what their goal was and successes and failures they have experienced. As you can imagine the reactions I have received from some of them right off the bat, especially the ones that we in earshot of their instructors. "You want me to say what I eat on a daily basis?" Yes, I had to reassure them that I would not share this information with their instructors and that it was all anonymous. I did tell them that I would be sharing it with you though, so sit back and get ready for the pain of others. Lol, Now I know this is supposed to be an inspirational book and all, but you should know me well enough by now that I can't start there. The first insert I need to use is from the first person that turned in her journal to me. She is a real sweetheart also I must say. She is in a couple of the classes I do at the Tamerac. She is 78 years old, I almost said young. I have to interject my first B.S. call of the book. I called her old not out ignorance but out of respect. We need to treat our elders with respect, they have earned it damnit why is that so hard for people to get through their thick heads. Sorry for my outburst, some things just strike a nerve when I hear them. Back to Ruthie, Ruthie like I said is a 78-year-old widow with a passion for life that I wish I could bottle up and pass it on to everyone who needs it. Ruthie reminds me a lot like Ms. Betty from Vegas, minus the happy hours. Lol She has a long history of health issues in her family. She explained in her journal that her Mother was the 14th of 14 children and all of her siblings were overweight and they all died from either heart attacks or strokes. That is horrible, Ruthie has been active her whole life trying to break the cycle set in motion by her family tree. She has two siblings her older brother became obese and died when he was 51 of a heart condition. Her younger sister had gastric bypass surgery but is still big and wheel chair ridden to this day. Ruthie did marry a career military man and lived together for 47 years, she said he was in great shape but just dropped dead one day, again horrible but like I stated in the last book tomorrow is not guaranteed. Her goal is to stay in the 140 range and eats and exercises daily. You noticed I said eats in all fairness I did say that I would not share this information with their instructors but for you all. All bets are off. So, I was perusing through Ruthie's entries and I came across an odd dinner selection, but without knowing the true intention behind it really didn't want to judge her on it. Like I said Ruthie journaled for a week, like I asked and out of courtesy to whoever took the time to fill out the journal I read them personally. So, Monday through Friday lunch everything looked very healthy. Then for dinner she ate three Almond Joy candy bars but they were the bite sized ones Lol I guess that makes it all good. Saturday was rainy and looks like she fell off the wagon because the only entry was ate more Almond Joy's she bought them for Halloween. lol I guess I know where I am going trick or treating, hopefully she restocks before then. She jumped back on the wagon Sunday and went back to her normal routine I am so glad for her, like I said she is a spit fire when she is working out. I can only hope to have half her energy if I have the privilege to live to be her age.

So, this brings me to my next ah ha moment, what makes us fall off the wagon? I know there can be a million reasons why, I guess the best advice I can give here is to be convicted to the reason you get back on the wagon. For Ruthie, her mission is to break the cycle of the road so many of her family members have gone down. She has already outlived almost all of them. I guess in a way she could have picked a more unhealthy menu choice to consume that rainy day. There are 90 calories in a bite sized Almond Joy. So, for three it was only 270 calories, I can't help her out on the nutritional value but I can give her a big hell yes, I love those damn things, so back in my fatter days I would have been right there with her, ripping away. Thank you, Ruthie, for your most excellent journal entries.

Bite sized- Bite Me: I missed the opportunity to call a big fat B.S. call last book on bite sized or fun sized candy bars. First, what's fun about bite sized candy? Like any fat person or skinny person that remained breathing after consuming the first one stopped at just one. You know it is unsatisfying when a skinny person eats just one and says "That's it?" Like I said before, I am a product of the sixties, next to Christmas, my friends and I lived for Halloween. We were probably the first group of teens to ever map out an entire community and place stars on all the houses that were must visit based on candy passed out in the past. The fun wasn't over when you got done with your three to four-hour bootie run, that was just when the physical activity part ended. After you made it to the dining room table with your pillow cases, yes cases with an S, and inspector 12 (Mom) searched your bags, you know for razors in apples, needles later in life, open packages, you know all the usual things, then it was time to catalog everything to our make shift inventory system that again wasn't invented back in the seventies before computers were even invented. I kick myself for not converting this early knowledge of spreadsheets into an app for today. But back then we were just protecting our treasures from our older siblings that were too cool to go out trick or treating, they would rather just cherry pick ours when we got home. Looking back today I feel like Smeagol in Lord of the Rings, "My Precious" when all the work was done and we got to dig into our full-sized candy bars. Getting back to the razor blade in the apples legend or myth? In all the years, I trick or treated I never uncovered a razor blade in any apples ever received. Just to be safe and to save time during the inspection process, my friends and I would dispose of any apples that we received as a treat. Think about it what kid in their right mind would choose an apple over a full-sized candy bar? Exactly said no fat kid ever!!! So usually we practiced our throwing skills for next little league season whenever we got an apple, just saying. One last tid bit before I move on, this falls under the trust issues I touched on last book. Kids see everything and even though we don't always call you out on it, we notice when your favorite candy never seems to pass inspection and it has to be held for further review and it is never seen again. Great job on hiding the wrappers from us though, good job. Ok, just so I don't have some health nut rolling up on me telling me the negative effects all that candy has on the fat assedy it brings to today's youth. I totally agree with you. The point I was trying to make is candy manufactures have taken the liberty to shrink down the size of this unhealthy product, while keeping the price about the same as it has always been and blaming it on the establishment for them having to create this lessor of a sized treat. It's all smoke and mirrors to me, just saying

Calories, Calories, look at all those little bastards!!! The calorie has to be one of a fat person's worst nightmare. They are everywhere food is, and the worst part is you can't see them you just know that they are there. This goes against every grain in my body, it's like when someone says to it's like that because that's the way it is. Or even better it's like that because it has always been like that. If you don't like the answer, ask a different question, or just do something different instead. Food manufactures have gotten very wise to the label readers as well as the fat people that just skim the labels and see what they want to see. Case in point, I mentioned in the first book about energy drinks, they have their place, I won't argue that but why are they hiding the true calorie count. Ok, by show of hands, honest hands, how many people have ever not drunk a full Gatorade 32 oz. thirst quencher on your own, in one sitting or even in a couple of big gulps? Exactly so then why would it be necessary for them to put on the front of the bottle 80 calories per 12 oz. serving, then when you turn the bottle around it says 2.5 servings per bottle. So instead you just consumed 200 calories in a couple gulps. Who gives a rip right? You should, the daily recommended calorie intake suggests a 2000 diet to be the most healthy. So now it's time to put on your oversized thinking caps. Sharpen up those pencils and crunch some numbers. Feel free to call Bull Shit anytime you want, I spent 10 years in banking but we were not allowed to add or subtract anything without the computers help. So, for today's lesson class, I have employed Cortana to conduct my food calorie searches on my brain box thingy here. I will give you the menu choice of one of the folks that submitted a journal and we can show a regular day of a healthy person and I will do a day in the life of me in the past. The healthy person will be played by Ruthie, since I have her journal handy.

Thursday Sept. 24 2016   Calories:

Breakfast: bowl of Kashi Cereal with 2% milk.   206 with milk
Lunch: 2 salmon patties 191 calories X2= 382   382
   ½ cup rice with broccoli   = 125   125
   ½ cup peas   = 59   59
   Water to drink   =0
Dinner: a little dish of macaroni salad we will say a cup. = 358   358
   No snacks added for this day   total:
               1033 for the day
Ok now it's my turn remember this was in my past and this is not the crazy me either this should be legitimate numbers.

Breakfast: Generic - 3 Fried Eggs, 4 Pieces of Bacon & 2 Slices of Whole Wheat Light Toast   491
Glass of oj   110
Snack 10 am bag of chips small   160
12 oz. can of soda   160
Lunch Burger King - Whopper Value Meal (With Cheese, Medium Fries, 946ml (32 oz.) Drink)   1430
Snack: snickers bar   250
Dinner: Spaghetti   280
    2 pieces of garlic bread   106
    Dinner salad with ranch   240
    2 x soda   320
Snack bowl of chocolate ice cream   267
          Total
          3863

Ok pencils down, this was a typical day in the life of this fat guy. No I didn't add in did you want to supersize this or jelly on the toast or coffee or dessert at lunch or if someone got laid last night and brought in doughnuts this morning. I'm sorry that was bad of me to say, but it's true. Fat people will use any excuse to bring treats into work and it's ok to eat them if someone brings them in to celebrate something in fact it's almost rude not to celebrate with them, isn't it? Hell, to the no it isn't!!! Just because they got laid, or had a birthday or had a child doesn't mean you need to add to your misery. Now if they bring in a healthy snack you could always substitute the one you were going to eat for the one they brought but under no circumstances should you eat both and blame it on them celebrating. That is a huge cop out. Ah Ha Moment, this week I had just hit my 100 pounds lost and I was joking about celebrating, my wife got off work a little early and I guess had a craving for pizza. She texts me and asked me what I wanted on my pizza, I promptly responded you text the wrong guy, because I don't eat regular pizza any more. Now she has been really supportive of my journey and maybe she thought I wanted to celebrate with some pizza. But that's almost like offering a recovering alcoholic a drink to celebrate his sobriety. Needless to say, the chicken stir fry I made when I got home was celebration enough for me and I thanked her for thinking about me though. Just a thought if you have someone you know on their own journey, never use food as a reward or punishment on them. It's not the foods fault for the shape we are in. It's the quantity of food and the times we put that food in our bodies. Before I finish with this section did you know a there are 3500 calories in a pound of fat. So even though they have been so gracious to offer us up 2000 calories as our daily recommended allowance you should want to know all the facts when you are deciding the healthy lifestyle menu choices you are considering. Just saying!!

Everybody's working for the weekend? Just like the songs says for everyone my age that knows who Loverboy is, "everybody's working for the weekend." Why is that? There are seven days in the week and five of them are during the week. We have two days that constitute the weekend, why do we focus just on those two days? I get it metaphorically those are typically our two days off for the week, if you are lucky enough to have a job that gives you weekends off. I am here to share another perspective with you though, for those of us that are disabled we don't go by a work week. Every day is special and every day is a work week for us too. For me other than going to church on Sunday, that's the only day I have to do anything out of my norm. So, I still have seven days to try to get healthy so maybe someday, but not today it might mean something more to me also. It drives me crazy though seeing the same faces everyday Monday through Friday working their ass's off to get to the weekend just to gorge themselves and start all over again on Monday. Here's a tip, why not try moderation on the weekend and maybe you wouldn't have to kill yourselves all week to still pay for the weekend. So here is my take on the weekends when it came to me and most guys when I was fatter. Ok so you did your 9-5 all week, now comes the weekend. Now depending what the calendar says on the wall determines what my weekend might look like. Let's make it easy and take this weekend for instance, since today is Friday. It is October 7, 2016 College football is in full swing so more than likely my Saturday will be spent taking in some football, what's watching football like having the buddies over and hanging out in the man cave? Can I get an Amen!! I'm sorry I mean a chest bump, I forgot my role in this scenario. I'm back, that also mean a trip to the grocery for the essentials right, beer check, pizza check, Doritos check, chicken wings check, brats check, beer check, got that already my bad, just got to be sure, that's just for me the guys will bring stuff too. Lol So Saturday morning comes got to eat a big breakfast so it soaks up the beer later, don't want to drink on an empty stomach, got to feel good tomorrow for NFL football. I forgot to mention that football is usually a two day event this time of the year and depending on who is playing that might mean a marathon of action, needless to say other than maybe going outside at half time and throwing the pigskin around that's the only physical activity going on this weekend other than the 12 oz. curls and if your wife has any interest in watching the guys run around in the tight pants too, then there may be some late night sports center going on if you know what I mean. Lol OK Fat guy get to the point it's almost kickoff!! My point is moderation!!! What's wrong with a couple of beers? Not a case, a couple of wings, not a dozen or 20, maybe skip the pizza one week, how about chips and salsa instead of nachos? All I am saying is cut back on the excess and oh ya Kick off is at 10am even on the pacific coast time, would it kill you to roll your ass out of bed a little earlier and maybe go for a walk before the game. Hey remember the body that carried your ass all week long at the grind and helped you earn the money for all the food you're about to devour over the next couple days? How about factoring a little me time into your touchdown celebration dance considering without me you would be nothing? Just saying, I guess the choice is yours, I could always order up a case of the squirts that would keep you on the throne for most of the first half if you would like also. It's your choice though, seriously.

What's wrong with this picture? So, what's wrong with this picture? We buy a new car, we baby it, we give it a bath when it is dirty, we try not to take it out of the garage when it is bad outside. We get it an oil change every 3000 miles, rotate its tires as well. If any of the warning lights come on we run back to the dealership and have it checked out. Why don't we do the same for our bodies? I know, I know I do that for my body too. Sure, you do, when was your last wellness exam? When was the last time you listened to it and actually did what you needed to do for it? Or did you do what all of us do and say I know what's best for it? And go about your day. The adage doesn't apply to if it ain't broken why fix it when it comes to your body. If you wait till its broken before you fix it, it might end up too late by that time. I know fat guy, go ahead try to scare me into working out, you forget by this time in the process you have already purchased the book or someone that loves you or thinks you need the motivation has purchased it. So, one way or another I'm getting paid so it's no skin off my fat ass weather you listen to me or not. All I am saying is why do we worry more about our car, more than we do about our bodies? I get it besides your house, your car is your next biggest expense and if you don't take care of it, how will you get to work? Exactly my point if you don't take care of your body the rest of it is a moot point. I failed to mention in the last book, my surgery and extended hospital stay at Mary Free Bed, was over $250,000 so unless you're driving a Lamborghini? You might want to adjust your priorities. Just saying.

The best things in life aren't Things? I think the Beatles might have been tripping a bit when they sang the lyrics "the best things in life are free." Everything costs and yes, the song does go on to say they want money. Money makes the world go around, no it won't buy happiness but it can help. One of the cruelest things I have had to deal with since having the stroke is watching everything I built crumble before my eyes. Proball Training Academy and Proball Arena were dreams of mine since I ever got involved in coaching sports. I always wanted my own training facility to help train and nurture young athletes to be the best they could be. I mentioned the hospital costs in the last chapter and the effects of what it costs to have a stroke. What price tag do you put on your dreams and your passion? It's hard to fathom until it is gone. I had hundreds of ball players that relied on me to get them ready every year for their season. My organization helped get several ball players college scholarships. So, to have that taken away because I couldn't take care of it anymore was devastating. No I am not saying that if you don't get yourself healthy you are going to suffer the same fate as I did, but statistics show that overweight unhealthy people live much shorter lives than fit, healthy people do. The reason I feel so compelled to continue on my journey and see this until the end, is to help the people that feel hopeless and to prove that it is never too late to choose life. The biggest ah ha take away for me on everything that has happened to me in my lifetime, is yes, money is important but the things we hold important in life money can't buy. Family, friends, and LOVE!!

Change your stars? Have you ever seen the movie "A knight's tale?" It's a movie with Heath Ledger, where a boy from a poor family is given to a knight to go on the road and be one of his servants as he travels the lands back in the days of jousting and medieval games. That is the premise of the story. The true meaning of the story is the father knows that for his son to have a chance at life he needs to change his surroundings and change his stars to be successful in life. Yes, I know this is a metaphor and yes, it's just a movie, but how many times have you seen a movie that has inspired you to do something good or different. Remember this book is about me, and I have. Movies like "The Blind Side", "Rudy", "The Rookie", "Rocky" ok even I can call B.S. on Rocky that was a totally made up fiction based movie, but who was Sylvester Stallone before the Rocky movies? Did you know he wrote the stories and almost didn't get cast in them? How would that have played out for him? Now he is one of the biggest stars in Hollywood. Ok fat guy get to the point!! Sometimes you have to leave your comforts of your surroundings and take a journey outside your comfort zone or circle of friends and family to get healthy. My trip to Nevada has turned out to be a life changing event for me, more than I ever expected. It has not just been about the weight loss or the improvement of my overall health, it has given me clarity on so many aspects of my life. It has proved to me how strong I am and not just in a physical way but mentally and spiritually. It has helped me get right with God and with family. It has gotten me to help eliminate the word can't from my vocabulary as well as to open up the horizons for my taste buds and try new healthy and exciting food choices. Could I have done this if I wouldn't have taken the opportunity and chance I was given 104 days ago, I have had 18,628 days in my 51 years of life so far, I don't know, you tell me. Change your stars!!

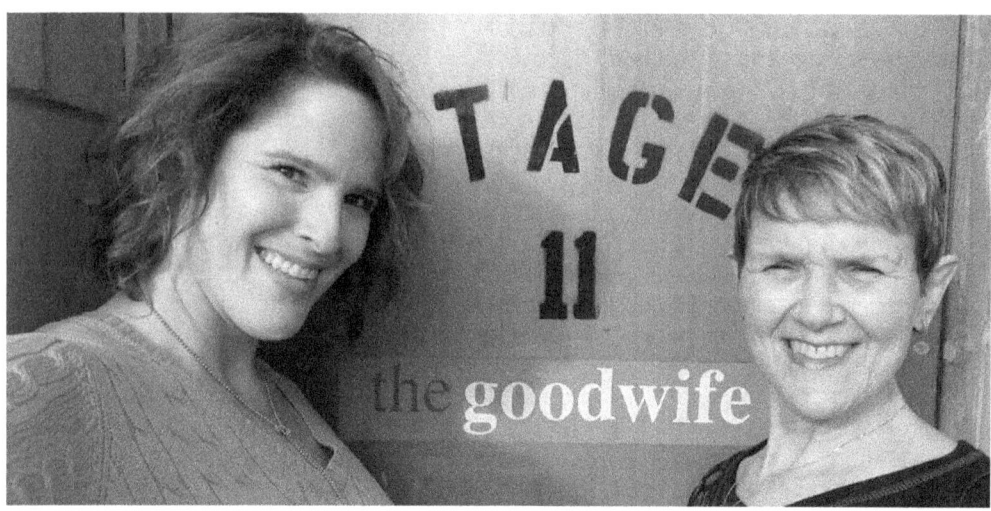

I have a niece Emily that is a great example of this. Emily comes from a single parent household of many years. She had a pretty shaky childhood but had a mother that loved her very much. Just when things were starting to get a bit normal for her, tragedy struck and her brother Jimmy was killed in a freak accident. That death affected my entire family. I come from a very large family, nine brothers and sister, 29 nieces and nephews, and a dozen or so great nieces and nephews. We have been fortunate enough to have only lost my parents and Jimmy so far. I was in my early 20's when we lost him, Emily was in her early teens and they were very close, she has had many opportunities to give up, yet she has continued to thrive. Her mother Linda is my oldest sister. She was the first one in my family to undergo stomach bypass over 20 years ago, She has probably been on the upside of that battle over the past seven years or so. Ok back to Emily, upon graduation, Emily went into the cosmetology field and started earning a living cutting hair. From there she pursued a career in plus size modeling in New York City. While in New York she landed some great jobs styling hair on a couple of little known shows like, Days of our Lives, The Tonight Show, The Good Wife, and her latest endeavor Brain Dead on CBS. She has traveled the world and lives life on her own terms. To say we are proud of her is an understatement of the fattest proportion. The last pictures I have posted in the beginning of the book were the day before I left for Vegas, at Linda's 65th birthday party. Here are just a couple of pictures of how fabulous she turned out.

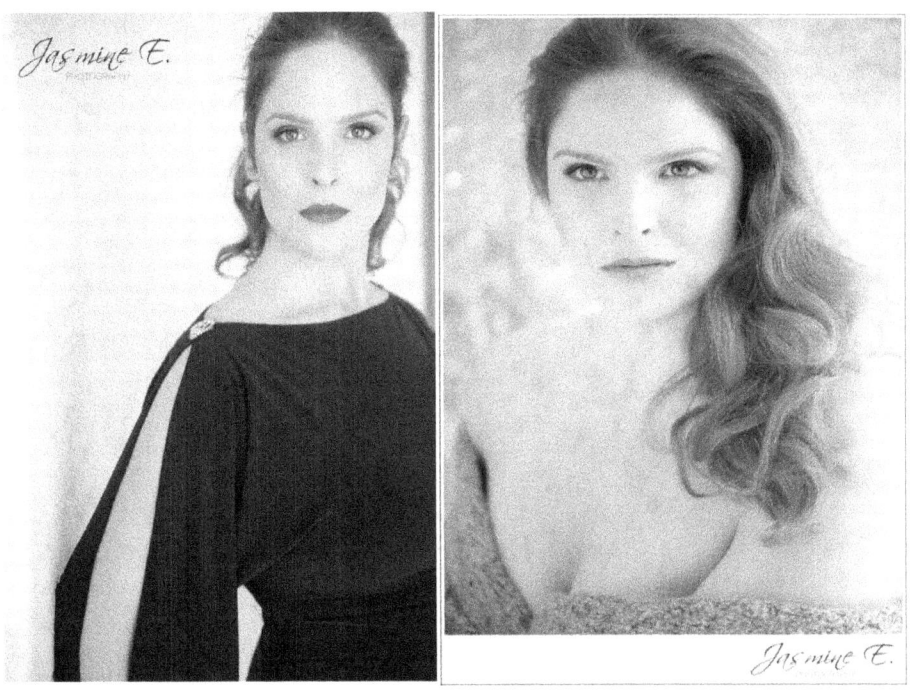

Jasmine E.

Jasmine E.

Gramma knows best? I know it's supposed to be "Mother knows best" but for this rant I need to use Gramma as the leading role. So, when it comes to baking and cooking great meals or if you need advice from someone that's been there she's your gal. Even when it comes to giving you medical advice, who do you think your mother learned it from? OK so here is where I call B.S. when I have an older than me product of the 30's 40's or 50's try to teach me about technology, that's where I draw the line. I know, if you spent the last 40 or so years in the technology industry, you are the exception to the rule. But if you have downed an apron over a sweater with your hair in a bun cooking up delicious treats for your grandchildren. It is you I am referring too. So, I am in the hot tub this morning before I hit the pool to start my workout and I set the timer for six minutes because I was on a time crunch today. I am in the tub working the hand weights getting my credit from my Garmin. The timer expires on the jets before I got my 5,000 steps in, just about then a nice older lady was about to get into the hot tub, she asked me if I wanted the jets on, I explain to her that I was almost done, but if she would like them on then that would be fine. She got into the tub as I was getting out she asked if I could add five minutes to the timer. I said of course, but like every thorough person of the older generation, she followed me to the timer and told me I wasn't doing it right when I put the timer on the five for five minutes. She explained to me that I had to turn the dial all the way to the end, then back it up to the five for that to be correct. Again, I call B.S. being the smart ass that I am, I had to ask why she did it that way and she gave me the standard old person response, "because that's the way I was taught to do it so that's the way it has always been." lol So that put my mind in motion, are we doomed to always be fat because if that's the way it has always been, why try to change now? Think about it, I blamed my parents in the last book for my fatness, when the real culprits were their parents and they can blame their parents and so on and so on. Right. That's why I didn't prosecute them in the first place, plausible deniability would be their defense. Lol While we are on the senior technology subject. I have a funny story to bust my Dad on. My Dad could pretty much fix anything with a matchstick, bottle of glue and duct tape. He was a MacGyver type guy of his generation. So, one Christmas back in the 80's, back when people still used VCR'S we bought him one. After a couple of hours setting it up for him we thought we had it figured out. NOT! About a week later I stopped by for a visit and noticed there was a piece of black tape on the front of the VCR. I quickly asked what had happened to it requiring the tape. My Dad quickly responded, "I got tired of seeing that damn 12 flashing at me so I fixed it." Lol For all of you that remember the VCR days, you should appreciate that one. Ok fat guy what does that have to do with weight loss? Nothing other than when you see a problem in your life, fix it! The faster you get it fixed the less irritation or downtime you will experience in the long run. Plus, just because it has always been done that way in the past, doesn't mean that's the only way to do it. I challenge you to fix yourself, while there is still time for fixing.

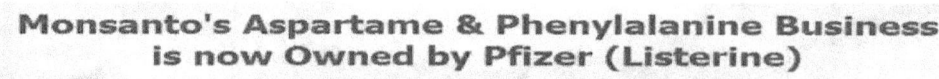

Monsanto's Aspartame & Phenylalanine Business is now Owned by Pfizer (Listerine)

WARNING: NEVER DRINK ASPARTAME !
NUTRASWEET, EQUAL, CREATINE, nor CANDEREL

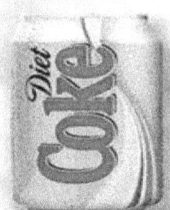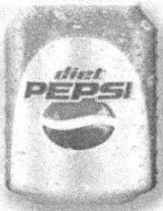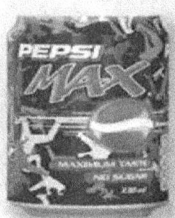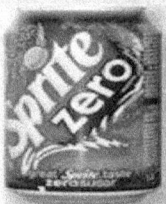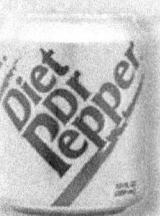

Just like fluoridated water, aspartame is literally a **poison in almost ALL of our food**. Aspartame causes seizures, brain tumors, multiple sclerosis (MS), and Grave's disease. In 1970, scientists fed milk with aspartame to 7 monkeys to study the effects. The final results: starting after 218 days - 5 monkeys had grand mal seizures and 1 died. **IT'S IN ALMOST ALL OF OUR FOOD!** Ever heard of Equal, NutraSweet, Creatine, or Canderel?

The deadly artificial sweetener nutrasweet is produced by feeding **fossil fuel OIL** to ecoli that are genetically modified to **DEFECATE** aspartame as **feces**. Not so sweet after you realize what you're actually eating!

Watch what you put in your mouth!!! I'm going to have to apologize in advance for this section. I am assuming that we are all adults here, I will try to keep it as PG as possible but I know I would be 50 shades of red if I was reading this to my Mother. With that being said, here we go. How many of us actually look at the food that we shovel down our gully's? Sure, we know what it is supposed to be when we order a number two combo, but do we really know what that meal is made out of? It's kinda like a hot dog, no two hot dogs are the same, the manufacturer lists the ingredients that they are made of, but not really sure how much of what are in each dog, right? Remember the part of the last book when I talked about choices? This chapter expands on that, for every choice we make there is a result from that choice, some good some bad. Like I said before no one was ever asked as a child what would you like to be when you grow up and the answer be "fat." So, let's take it a step further and this is where we get older, if 80% of weight loss is nutrition and 20% is exercise, why don't we pay more attention to what goes in our mouths? For this scenario, I will be playing the part of the guy and since I don't have any immediate friends that are prostitutes, I will have to make one up, we will call her Trixie. I am assuming here that when a young lady is asked when she is young, what would she like to be when she grows up a prostitute is pretty low on the list of choices. Yet remember I just left the state of Nevada where prostitution is legal and for some of them they make a good amount of money doing it, no pun intended. So, let's drill down even deeper into this question, if you gave a prostitute the choice of what she wanted to put in her mouth, you could probably guess what she didn't want in it. Then why do we continue to put unhealthy food into ours? There are thousands of choices available out there for us, but a Twinkie is what we chose? Really Remember the part in segment one that I talked about taking a natural product and covering it or adding toppings and sauces or dressings to it and making it unhealthy? Keeping with the adult theme, this is the best way I can break this down for you through this fat guys eyes. Oral sex, if you survey 100 men and ask them how many like oral sex 99 will say yes and there will be one liar. With women, you would probably get a 50/50 response 50% that like it and 50% that have never had it done right to them. Just saying. Getting back to the example of the 99 men that didn't lie, if you asked then how many need extras to enjoy oral sex such as chocolate sauce, whipped cream, jellies. 98 of them would say they didn't care about using them and you got it one more liar. If you ask the ladies I am guessing 50/50 again, 50% would like the added treat, the other 50% know they would get left with the cleanup and it wasn't worth the mess. The moral of the story is why take a natural act that can be calorie free and have such a positive impact on a person as oral sex and make it unhealthy by adding un needed calories and mess for the same amount of pleasure? For this scenario, Trixie was definitely not for kids. LOL

Bypass this!!! When will we learn, there is no miracle cure for fatness? Yes. gastric bypass will make us conform to a regiment unless you enjoy the dumping process of the procedure? Unfortunately, I have known as many people that this procedure didn't work for, the ones it did work for. Does that make me an expert on it? No, but as a fat person, living in a fat person's world a lot of my friends live in this same world to. I know that it is a long process to get to the part of the surgery. For some it takes over a year to get to the surgery. I know you have to go to counseling prior to surgery and they have support groups after surgery to help you cope with the changes. I know it's a double-edged sword, trying to teach a fat person how to eat like a skinny person while they are still fat. We can't grasp the concept of eating like a bird when we are used to eating an ostrich.The other thing people forget is the stomach is an organ that will stretch and in many cases, stretch to the size it was before surgery and bigger. Without committing to the complete lifestyle change, you are setting yourself too tough and long road of pain and misery. Don't get me wrong, for some people this is their last-ditch effort such as mine was, I pray to God it works for you. I just asked Cortana about the failure rate and she said it's between 40 & 60% of gastric bypass patients fail but those numbers fall back on the patient not the doctors performing the surgery. People again think that this is their miracle cure. Go in snip snip, put the band on and away we go. B.S. your body still has its cravings, it still is accustomed to its portion size and it will find a way to get satisfied no matter how many times you get sick in the process. Remember I had three siblings go through it, my oldest sister after years has beat the system and learned to live healthy. My second oldest sister was the last one to do the surgery and has seen little result and my older brother, has had multiple heart issues after his surgery that has helped him have to stay on a regiment to stay healthy.

Food is a horrible drug!!! I am sure this next rant is going to strike a nerve for many of the establishment type folks out there as well as people in the medical world, but again this is weight loss through the eyes of this fat guy. Thank God, I live in a country where the freedom of speech is still protected. Rant locked and loaded sir!! You thought Big Pharm. Was our biggest problem, how can we see the forest through the trees when it comes to our food choices? No I don't mean healthy food choices, or do I? We live in the greatest country on earth, Yes, I know it is debatable sometimes, but for this fat guy, there is no place I would rather be then the U.S. of A. We live in the world of free enterprise and with that brings the endless supply of choices. Really how many variety of candy bars do we actually need and why are they always located in a place where you are bored out of your mind waiting in line to check out and can't wait to get to your car and rip open your box of Twinkies? Can I get a high five!! So instead you rationalize the nutritional value between the king-sized snickers staring you in the hairy eyeball, or the Twinkie that has an endless shelf life, but is likewise delish!! Then you make the adult like executive decision, I will choose the king-sized Snicker bar because it won't hurt to put the Twinkie's on the shelf for the one or two days depending how many mouths you have in your household to consume that box and I will eat my precious in the car or at the checkout as soon as I feel safe that my debit card isn't going to be declined. Don't lie to me fat people, we have all been there. Talking about the debit card decline. No one would ever rationalize the choice between a Snickers and a Twinkie, they are two different food groups, right? Snickers is a candy and a Twinkie is a bread so it's all good, look it up on that pyramid thingy I am sure they taught us that back in school somewhere. I know that's the lighter side to the real problem facing fat people today, so many choices so little time. Obesity is a national epidemic; it leads to more deaths than every other cause of death known to mankind. Wait a minute fat guy do you have proof of that. No, remember I am just a fat guy spewing my rants, but remember I do have a history of being fat and even though I only hear out of one ear now since the surgery God has still blessed me with two eyes and the ability to hear pretty damned good out of my right ear. Obesity is one of the main causes for the following according to the National Heart, Lung, and Blood Institute. So, if obesity is one of the main causes of heart disease, stroke, cancer, hypertension, diabetes and so on and so on. How could it not be considered a pandemic colossal reason to help control fat people syndrome? Easy, food is not an illegal substance. Everything out of moderation has the potential to kill you, should we put a ban on everything? The FDA's job is to regulate what a manufacturer puts on a label is actually what it is. They also try to monitor that food is kept free of poisons and are stored at the proper temperatures so we don't die of an immediate death, but remember the goal of any business is to not kill its customers quickly right.

If they get 20 or 30 years of your money they win, right? So, what are you saying fat guy? Big brother needs more regulations to save us from ourselves? No wise ass, I am saying we need to start saving ourselves from ourselves. I will be one of the first to scream B.S. if anyone wants to blame the government for us being fat. All I want from the government is to make sure the manufacturers post the correct information on the packaging. Stop allowing them to slick talk us into thinking that it's ok to eat a million-calorie product without knowing how bad it really is for us. Didn't they do that with the cigarette companies and look how much that did for us? I agree a warning label of the side of a snickers bar is not the answer, remember most fat people don't read past the giant SNICKERS on the front of the candy bar. The only way I see the situation of obesity to get better is keep your mouth shut. No I don't mean stop talking about the problem, I mean stop eating the problem. Start focusing on eating healthy and leave the empty or bad calorie foods on the shelf. That doesn't mean that you go back in a couple of weeks and buy them at a discount because they have marked them down because their expiration date is fast approaching, remember a Twinkie has like a 50-year shelf life. I am saying treat everything like a Twinkie, put all the crap on proverbial shelf and don't touch it for 50 years, if you still want it 50 years from now, God willing we are still on this planet then eat away. Just saying the choice is yours.

Good to the last drop: As a product of the 60's, jingles have played a big part of my life. Then again some of them shape our habits as we grow up too. I am a firm believer in the term "waste not want not." and being from the 60s I grew up with a lot of people that lived through the great depression. I also believe that many of the food habits we still use come from generations before us. Fat Camp Test, show of spatulas, how many of us throw out anything without using a spatula to get out every last ounce of goodness left in the container. Why… because we were always told don't waste food right. Again, I am not suggesting wasting anything, but we need no break the cycle of worrying about wasting food and eating more of it so we don't waste it. One of the ongoing fights I had with my sister at fat camp was her constant bitching about leftovers. I would prepare good healthy menu items every night pretty much and then focus on portion control and restraint during dinner, so inevitably there would be left overs after every dinner, mostly because I hadn't learned or reconditioned myself to cook lesser amounts of food. So, we would wrap the food up in Tupperware and stick it in the fridge. Right? So, I forgot to tell you earlier Alzheimer's runs in my family. It never failed by about Wednesday when I would get ready to cook dinner, my sister would look in the fridge and start a fight because there were all these left over's going to waste and I was cooking something new. Remember by this point I was on my daily regimen. I had my usual first meal of the day, then I would do a smoothie for my second meal and then a normal healthy third meal. It really left me anytime to eat left overs. Believe me, I am never too good to eat left overs, I am the product of a Mother that could reinvent several nights of leftovers into a gourmet meal like we had never experienced in our lifetime. Lol and a Dad that would say keep your damn mouth shut and just eat it. Hahahahah So why is it so hard to break the chain of wasting food, or taking less because we feel we need to eat until we are past full? Trust! the fear of the unknown. We get these thoughts instilled in us from conceptions basically. What if? What if the power goes out how will we cook dinner? What if we don't eat it all now? Will someone else eat our portion? What if we run out of money and can't buy food? What if what if, what if? Trust!!! What if this were to happen? Think of the solution before you pound down the extra food. Why do I need that extra helping of food? If it makes sense, then do it. If it's just because I'm a grown ass man and I said so, you might want to rethink that answer. Put the spatula down if the answer is I don't need any more than I already have in my dish. Heaping your dish just to not waste what is in the bottom of the jar is not the right answer. Just Saying.

Are you still hungry? Or did it just taste good? Have you ever reached for seconds at meal time and wonder why the hell you are doing that? Are you still hungry, or is it the fact that it tastes so damn good you wanted more of that deliciousness? One thing you need to remember is it takes on average 20 minutes for your body to register that you are full. So, if you are a fat person like me that eats in lightning speed, are you still hungry or? This is a tricky doubled edged sword for me. I try my hardest to only eat what I put on my plate the first time I sit down to eat. I rarely take any seconds, unless I have workout extra hard that day and if for some reason, I missed a meal time. It does happen from time to time. If I can avoid eating more, then I know I would benefit from not making up for the missed portion, but remember the trust issues you will create with your body, if you try to starve it? Sometimes less is less in the grand scheme of things. If you take in less calories than your body requires it will go into a hoarding mode and you will actually gain weight. So, achieving the proper balance with your body is key. I cannot tell you what that balance is for you. I only know what my balance is. My body is quick to point things out to me if it doesn't like what I am doing to it. For example, I am super focused on losing weight, so the scale is my worst best friend. I tend to hang on every number change or balance of the scale. My body knows this also, so it seems whenever I start eating less each week I am in this challenge, my body gives up less and less weight. It doesn't seem to matter how much exercise I do in conjunction with my intake for that week. Last week I worked out half the week and ate much more than I ate the previous week and I lost five pounds last week and six lbs. The week before, we will see how week three goes and compare the results then.

Silence is golden!!! So, I just got back from the gym and I am irritated so please forgive my rant. You ever hear the phrase "silence is Golden?" The gym should be a pretty serene place, no not as quiet as a library. But nothing pisses me off as much as a Guido grunting and hooting and hollering because he just maxed out twice. Dude if I want to hear grunting I will record my pre-workout dumping ritual. Hearing you act like you are giving birth to triplets all at once every time you push a weight up and down ain't getting it for me or any of the other senior citizens working out around you. If you are so proud of your accomplishments, they make something for you it's called a home gym. Clear a couple of folding chairs out of your man cave/ basement and grunt away. While I'm pissing off all the meat heads at the gym, roid man, yes you the one that is pacing around with a death face on, trying to psych yourself up so you can do your three reps. The weights are your friend, what have they ever done for you that you find it necessary to throw them around after each time you use them? Again, it's just an inanimate object, it has never done anything to you or said your baby's ugly or anything. Here's a thought cut back on the roids and work out like a normal person, Bodybuilders R Us, called they are going to pass on your membership into their hall of fame, sorry. One more for you, weigh me guy, if you think every time you do a set of something your weight is going to change? Obviously, you have watched too many Popeye episodes where he eats the spinach and his arms get huge. It's a cartoon dude, not sure what you're looking to reveal by stepping on the scale every five minutes but it ain't gonna happen, sorry! Just saying.

Are we there yet? You know you have asked it before, we are all little kids, riding it a car towards vacation. Are we there yet? Remember life like weight loss is a journey not a destination. Only you can answer that question are you there yet? How do you feel; no seriously how do you feel? If the answer is just ok, you're not there yet. Doctors have been so gracious to put together some B.S. chart that lumps everyone together and tells them what is best for them. Sorry Doc. I will tell me how I am feeling, how about I rely on you to tell me what's wrong with me when I am sick. Deal? Fat people, skinny people, old people young people die. This is just the nature of the beast, how we live is what should really matter. If you like feeling like crap, keep doing what you're doing, you obviously have mastered this move. When you decide, there is more to life than just getting by, take the reins, and drive your own sleigh for a change. No before the B.S. Chants start. Did I say anywhere that this was going to be easy? Nothing in life that is good, is easy? If it was easy we would all be in perfect condition, right? Instead if you are reading this book or an overachieving skinny person you have figured out you need to make a lifestyle change. Congratulations, you have taken the first step to your journey. Admitting you have a problem is the first stem in most programs. Just being fat doesn't qualify you to join this club. You need to realize that you have a problem that needs to be fixed. Remember the part where I said I didn't have an eating problem, I see food and I eat it no problem. That's what I am talking about. If you see food and can't not eat it, therein lies the problem. Baby steps, until you can hit your groove and find your happy place. Trust me I never thought I could do what I did the past 105 days. I left for Nevada and had the opportunity to donate all the clothes I had in my closet to charity if I thought I was going to lose all this weight. I came home to a closet and a dresser full of cloths that are too big for me except for the 2 xl's that I bought and could never wear because they were too small. So, are we there yet? For me no, I have set a goal of another 100 lbs. Then I still won't be there yet. I won't be there till they put me in the ground, remember life is a journey not a destination. I want to be in control of my journey. God Speed on yours.

A pound is a pound. Damnit!! Have you ever heard the riddle "if you dropped a pound of gold or a pound of feathers off the empire state building, which will hit the ground first? If the theory of gravity is correct they should hit at the same time, because a pound is a pound. So how come it is whenever you hit a plateau, the first thing out of most trainer's mouths is "did you know muscle weighs more than fat?" What does that have to do with the price of tea in China? A pound of fat should weigh the same is a pound of muscle, Right? I don't want to hear that I worked my ass off all last week and since I transferred fat and built muscle that is why I didn't see a weight loss. I will be the first to call B.S. on that. For example, I weighed in last Tuesday at 300 on the nose, I knew I needed to weigh in for the next challenge later that day, So I did what every other fat guy faced with another competition would do and started drinking water. Remember one gallon of water equals eight pounds and this is a zero-calorie product, so hell yes, I drank like a fish. You need to remember I am starting a fresh challenge after just losing 100 lbs. No, I am not getting any credit for the weight I just lost. So, I figured why give my competition a free 100 lbs. So, I drank and drank and drank. I May even have stayed away from the bathroom until I weighed in also, no living proof of that, no cameras in there. Lol So I weighed in later that afternoon at 316.5 needless to say I wasn't happy to see the scale go up, but I took one for the team so to speak, because this is a two-person challenge. I am teamed up with my physical therapist. So, I figured no blood no foul, right? I would just work my butt off to cut the water weight and be back on track, this Tuesday. Well they must have gotten wind of my dastardly plan, because I had to re weigh in Wednesday and have my body measurements recorded. I weighed in at 315.0 Wednesday morning. Since Wednesday morning, I have done six Tabata exercise classes, three energizer classes and one spinning class as well as all of my regular daily workouts and about 20 trips to the sauna. Still after all that I weighed in at 304, when I left the Tamerac today. That's still 11 lbs. Lost in a week, I guess I should be happy with that, but I am not. If I was at 289 I would be, but that won't be the case tomorrow. So, I started reviewing other reasons I might not have lost as much weight as I thought I should and I realized that I have eaten more food this past week then I am accustomed to. I see that I have been eating more second meals, then just doing cabbage or an energy bar. I know I have been working out a lot more, I don't know if I can say more, but definitely differently. That could explain my increased appetite, the weather is getting colder also, so that might be playing a factor also. I am glad that I am journaling not only my fitness, but my nutrition also, the journal is a good reference point when you question why you aren't getting the results you are expecting. So, the moral of this rant, is don't get discouraged if you don't see a weight loss every week. If you question the numbers, look back at your activities and intake and see if that's your issue. Never rule out operator error either. Weigh yourself again if that makes you feel better, try another scale. Just don't settle with being disappointed. If all else fails, change up your routine, shake it up, your body may be getting bored and a change may do you good.

Community pool? Get with it people. Some people don't grasp the concept of community property; it makes me shake my head. There is a big difference between public and private, public is everyone's private is yours. So, one of the knock I had on the Tamerac, the gym I worked out at was the music they played over their overhead sound system. I realize the clientele was an older group, but there is something lacking in motivation when you are trying to get moving to 60's & 70's classic rock, just saying. So, within the past week they started playing generic workout music, which was better. No, it's not the original artists but at least it is upbeat and motivating. So, that brings me to my boundaries rant. Here I am four hours deep into my workout, in the pool working away, minding my own business, in my own world got my jam going "Gloria" I believe. Don't judge! When all of a sudden, the music dies. LOL not actually but in reality, one of the older ladies walks out of the storage room where the volume control is housed for the pa. and made the executive decision that we were going quite for a while. Me being the quite conservative easy going person that I am, lost my shit a bit. Remember she was my elder, so I wasn't disrespectful but like I said it's my jam, but more important there were four of us in the pool at the time, who gave her the right to be the boss of us and decide that we needed the silence. Needless to say, the music came back to life really quick like. Moral of the story, when you are working out in a public facility, check with the other members before you make an executive decision that affects all involved. If you are the only one working out at the time, you have first choice on items you can chose, but when you are the last one to the party, it is always better to ask to do something, then to disrupt everyone else's mojo. Just saying

So, I shaved my ____ for this? So, it happened, I knew it was going to, I didn't know it was going to take five months for it to happen though. I gained two pounds last week. I weighed in today for the fall into fitness challenge and for week three, I gained two pounds. Wait for it, wait for it, Now. WTF!!!!!!! I had that feeling going into today, that something wasn't right. I woke up this morning at 4:03am, so that was good. I decided to shave my beard down, because it is pretty grey, ok I call bull shit, because I thought it would help. I got to the gym at 5:05 and quickly ran over to the scale in the locker room, for a pre-game check and that scale had me at the same weight as last week, so I knew I was screwed when I had to weigh in on the official scale out on the fitness floor, because that one is on carpet and two pounds heavier than the scale in the locker room. Sure, enough, I was at 306. Two pounds higher than last week. So, what do you do? I know what I wanted to do. My first thought was to run down to Wal-Mart and buy a family sized package of double stuffed Oreo's and a gallon of chocolate milk and dip my sorrows away. Next, would be line up my stuffed animals and send out the invitations for my pity party. What did I do? I did 20 mins in the sauna, 10 mins in the hot tub, did Kate's Tabata class, did my lower body workout, hit the hot tub and sauna, and started looking at my journals from last week. I realized that I didn't work out hard enough and I didn't eat enough good food for my body to continue to burn the fat I needed it to. I told the ladies at the desk, if they saw the two pounds I gained hanging around, tell it was looking for it and I was going to kick its ass. Lol Another thing I was hoping wouldn't bite me in the ass was my internet issue. I talked about this earlier. We are switching internet providers and there was a lapse in connections for the last week, so no big deal, I have been working on the book at the Tamerac, after my workouts of course. Well it seems I may have been doing too much typing and not enough working as well as working through my second meal of the day. I think those two things also contributed to the weight gain. So, live and learn, onward and upward. Damn, those Oreo's sounded good too!! Just saying.

Breaking tradition? One of the hardest things I have found for me since returning back to Michigan after the journey began in Vegas, is breaking traditions, traditions may be a strong word choice, but it is more than a habit and less than tradition let's say. You know how it is, it seems every time you do that certain something, something that you have always done in your life there seems to be a food associated with it. For example, whenever I go to the mall with my wife, she has to go in by Yonkers, no biggie right, wrong as soon as you exit Yonkers into mall, there is an Auntie Annie's Pretzels. Smelling delicious as always, I might add. This one is a no brainer, but it still is hard to pass up one, it is fall here in Michigan so it's time to go to the apple orchard, right? Apples aren't fattening, right? No but the cider and doughnuts and caramel apples that accompany them are. Lol My big test will come this weekend; I have broken my training regimen and headed to the north country to deer camp with my lifelong friend Christopher. We have been friends for 47 years and have hunted together for 35 years. So, over those years we have enjoyed some pretty good but not always so healthy of menu choices. I must say this year has been a bit different to say the least. Remember the last time I saw Chris was just prior to heading to Vegas, so that was 100 lbs. ago. It always seemed that we somehow always ended up with way more food than we ever needed. Lol I wonder why that happened? This year I packed the cooler up, with things I currently eat, raw cabbage, yogurt, granola, breakfast bars, fruit, and water. I even have to call B.S. on this one. What kind of hunter packs that way to go to a five-day deer hunting camp? I guess my answer would have to be the guy that want's a chance at continuing the tradition! You see only 107 days ago, I wasn't sure I would see another deer season and if I did, it would probably be my last. 36 seasons are a lot of seasons but 70 seasons, would be a lot better. I am a realist, I realize this could always be my last camp, we are not guaranteed another one. I need to make the most out of everyone I have the opportunity to have. But the healthier I get, the more chances I have at more deer camps, Right? By the way today is Ms. Betty's birthday. Happy Birthday!! On a side note, I need to expand on my buddy, Christopher. Chris and I met when he was four and I was three. I was in my driveway pounding nails into my driveway, he lived across the street from me and came over and asked if he could join in the fun. We have been best friends ever since. He has seen me at my best and he has seen me at my worst, yet through it all he has remained my best friend. My wife knows if I ever left her for anyone else, he would be that person. No, we are not gay, but if there is anyone out there that gets me as a person, Chris is the one. I think of everyone I have run into since being back from my first journey, Chris has been the most excited about my progress. Like I said he gets me, he knows I wasn't happy with myself 107 days ago, He never pushed me to lose weight, he supports me in any way he can though. He was there for two days during and after my brain surgery. He always makes me feel welcomed at his deer camp. He has even changed some of his deer camp rituals to do healthier meals for us while I am here. BTW Chis is about 6'3 145 lbs. soaking wet. He is from a strong Hungarian heritage. He eats a lot of hot spicy foods, and is a firm believer of at least one alcoholic beverage a day. You did notice the at least part, I am sure that he and Jim Beam have had more than one a day for many a day. Lol He also believes that everything in moderation and that weight loss is a lifestyle change not a diet. He is another big reason I fight to be alive.

Congratulations on achieving the BIG O!!! NOT!!!! We should be excited, Right? We are now officially obese Today's society has given us our own classification. Many of us have dreamed about our first big O, I bet you never thought it would be obesity? So now what do we do? Start blaming everyone for what has happened too poor poor pitiful me? I guess you could do that, blame the government? Obama only has a couple more months in office, he would be an easy target. How about blaming the Keebler Elf? I am sure if you put your fat foot in front of the tree house door, so no more of the elves could come to his aid, we could probably beat his ass. Lol for real though what do we do? I don't know about you, but I chose life and started listening to what my body wanted. I made things simple for me, if my body didn't need it, then it doesn't get it. Sweets, no, pop, no, processed food, no, white flour, no. Basically if it was too high in sugar, salt or flour I do my best to eliminate it. Is it always possible, no, do I always look for alternatives to that product, yes? When it is, all said, and done, it doesn't matter how you got here, we all have a story and a million reasons why. The only thing that matters is how do we get ourselves out of this situation. In honor of our classification and since the mile-high club has already been taken. I have decided to create the "Big Sexy Obesity Association or "Big Sexy Obesity Ass. For short. To join you must complete the following pledge and send me (0) $'s but you do need to keep it somewhere that you can see it and use it as motivation to get yourself out of this club. Please send me the contract when you have reached your healthy goal weight so I can add you to my wall of fame.

Big Sexy Obesity Ass.

I, Name: _____, on Date, _____

Declare myself obese, by today's standards. It doesn't matter how I got to this point, the only thing that matters is that I get out. I will do everything in my power to get healthy for failure is not an option. I will use this contract to motivate me to stay on track. I will use it as have so many people just like me, to achieve my success to a healthier lifestyle. To everyone that has supported me up to this point in my journey, thank you very much, but for me, the next 10 words have to be my new best friends. "IF IT IS TOO BE, IT IS UP TO ME!!"

This is a matter of life or death. Mine.

Signed: _____,

God speed Love Big Sexy.

What age are we? I have said over and over, I am a product of the 60's, I am younger than the "Baby Boomers and younger than the "Depression age" or the Golden Oldies." I think I am too old to be a "Millennial "and thank God I am not a member of the "entitlement generation." Does that make me a member of generation "X" or even a member of the "Pepsi" generation? I guess in the long run it doesn't change who I am or what I am as long as I live my life according to works best for me. Society in general loves to make up cute titles to call people without ever considering what effect it might have on them. It is sad in a way that we just can't be the person that we were born to be without being stereotyped into a category to make some statistical numbers freak happy that everyone is accounted for, like who is counting anyway? You might be wondering where this rant is going? So, get to it fat guy!! Okay, so I was at the gym today sitting in the café area, typing on the book, when a mother and her son sat down at the table next to me. The mother was getting ready to drop her son off at the daycare the gym provides for its members. I couldn't help to notice that the boy was still in his pajamas, which was a little odd since it was 9:30 am but remember I don't judge. Just my luck on of her Millennial friends came over for a chat, so I got some good intel for the book. The mother ordered a double espresso from the café, while she ordered the son a Pop Tart, he was all good with the bug juice he was sipping on, I guess. As he fixated on the IPad he was watching I heard the mom explain to her friend that he was learning Spanish on the IPad. The program he was watching was designed to teach kids Spanish as they watched the program. Before you scream B.S. I kinda already figured that one out. Supposedly the program doesn't actually teach them this cool trick now that they are under five years of age, she explained to the other mother that, the process just subliminally stores the words they are learning in their sub conscious, until such time as they have Spanish class in school, then the words resonate with the child as if they have known them for years. Isn't that special? Trust me, it took all I could do not to scream out Bull Shit, but I controlled myself, instead I was trying to control my emotions about the child's nutritional habits being formed at that very moment. Kudos to the mom, for making the effort to get to the gym and work on your health, but a double espresso before you work out? That's a bit risky, isn't it? Then we have little Johnny or whatever his name was, learning Spanish at age four, because this is his most impressionable years, says the IPad program thingy, so let's teach him that it is ok to go to the gym in your pajamas, eat a pop tart and drink a bug juice. That covers about 0 of the daily recommended food groups. It almost nips the corner in one of the categories if you squint your eyes and stretch the truth a bit. The younger you teach your kids to eat healthy, the longer your child will eat healthier. That is a proven fact. Think about it, even if they only eat healthy while they live in your house, from 0-18, it would take until year 37 for them to eat unhealthier than when they lived with you and that is if they decided to go bat shit crazy for the 18 years after they moved out. See my point?

You know you can be to overprotective, right? II Remember the part where I am not Dr. Phil, nor am I Dr. Seuss. I am just a fat guy, with years of experience being fat and a ton of nieces and nephews and great nieces and nephews. My oldest nephew is 46, and my youngest niece is eight. So, I run the gamut on experience there too. This rant will be brief, because every parent has their own parenting philosophy and the fact that when you try to interject your own personal philosophies when they are not asked for, panties get in a bunch. So, most of the time I just sit back and watch the action. You know the do as I say not as I do theory of parenting, doesn't really work, right? Maybe it does when they are in front of you, but get them alone, with their cousins and if these walls could talk, begins. Where do you think the phrase "chip off the old block" and "the apple doesn't fall that far from the tree." Or even "Why doesn't your family tree branch?" I apologize for that one, remember I live in the sticks and I digress. Getting back to your kids, they don't miss anything, you may think they don't know your little secrets, but trust me, they are just working on the angles to see when they can use them against you for their biggest bang for the buck. Case in point, one Sunday dinner, my in-laws we up from down state, we were just wrapping things up and my oldest daughter, being about nine at the time, pipes up with I know what the "F" word means. Being shocked that she even brought that up in the first place and in the company of my in-laws was horrific for myself and my wife. So, we did what every other good Christian parent would do and said, Andrea, I think you must be mistaken. Unfortunately for me she said no, mother. "daddy says it all the time when he is mad." Needless to say, neither her or I had any dessert that evening. Kids say the darndest things. Lol I have another niece that has been sheltered from soda, and sweets pretty much her entire life. That is a great thing in theory, but wait until she starts getting her freedom and venturing out with her friends. This is where the fat hits the fan. How quick will it be before she discovers the many flavors of unhealthy food choices awaiting her. Sure, the words sugar overload come to mind, but in my mind so does the resentment from her on her parents from keeping these secrets from her for so long. That's why I am so pro in moderation. Give your kids the real thing but offer them the healthy choice as well and guide them from there. If we try to control them while they are under our control, there is a better chance of them being out of control when they are on their own. Love them for all that they are and guide them to all they can be…

See you in my dreams. You ever have those days, when your mind goes on overload and it seems you're like some fat philosopher or something like that? I don't know if I am having one of those days or not, or if it is all the Ibuprofen I am on from the root canal I had yesterday. Anyway, here goes anyway. I talk a lot about journey and changes and going, forward right? All of us have people in our lives that always live in the past. They constantly remind us of our past. That can be a good thing but most of the time as a fat person, I would rather visualize my future and where I want to get. Our history is a great reminder of where you have been and what got you to today, but it also has a tendency to hold us back also. I have decided as of 5:26am 10/21/16 that just because you are a part of my history, if you can't or won't leave our past in the past. You won't be a part of my future. I won't allow you to take me off my journey, because you are stuck in the past. I hope that doesn't make me sound like a jerk, but I feel the effects of how this tares at my heart and affects my motivation. Unfortunately, it is usually a family member that I am talking about. This doesn't mean you don't love them or that they won't still be a part of your life going forward. It just means that going forward, they won't be as big a part of your future as maybe they had been in your past. Remember yesterday is history, tomorrow is a mystery and today is a present given to you from God. We can't change our past, but we can change our future. I will always have you in my dreams, even if I don't have you in my future. Just saying. Stay the course. So,unfortunately, I received word today from my sister Donna today, that she has entered Hospice care. She doesn't expect to make three weeks; I have a hard time processing that information. Knowing the power of the mind and the wonderful things it can do for you and against you. I would have hoped she could have chosen to fight longer. I told her that I would support her decision and love her forever and this little poem popped into my head and heart for her.

I will not mourn your passing, I will not shed a tear,

your memories surround me, you're voice I'll always hear.

Until the day we meet again, my heart will skip a beat,

until my lovely sister, again, our hearts will meet.

I will always love you more Sis!!!

My Sister Donna passed away the evening of, December 2nd, 2016. one day before the three year anniversary of my stroke. To say that my inspiration is gone, would be an understatement. I have so much more to live for now that I am in a healthier state but it still hurts down to my soul, to lose someone that was in the fight for health as much as I was. I will always love her and appreciate her motivation, that she inspired me with. Love you Sis.

Can't see the forest for the trees! I just had an ah ha moment. As I sit here in my hunting shack typing on my computer, I never really thought about it but my hunting shack has four windows. Yes, you might be thinking that's pretty standard fat guy. It's so you can see all around you. Wait for it, wait for it no B.S, but I generally only look out the main window where I have my best shot at the deer. The other three are not the most optimal shots to be taken, especially with a crossbow. But yet there is still a chance that I am missing an opportunity if I don't look out them. Let me break it down for you, for any hunters out there. I shoot my crossbow left handed, so the first widow to my right is the main window I look out of. I really never pay attention to the other three, because the chances of getting a good shot out of those windows are much less. Does it mean that it is impossible to shoot out them? No, it just means that I would prefer to shoot out of my main window. Case in point, when you are faced with a problem, that one, you are unfamiliar with or not in your comfort zone. Don't dismiss it as not achievable unless you try to achieve it at least three times. The good ol college try of once, is long gone, science has proven that it usually takes 21 tries to form a habit. For me it makes me wonder how many more deer I might have seen if I was looking out all my windows. I harvested this 10-point buck out my left blind window opening day 2016. I had to shoot opposite handed to get him. Nothing is impossible... Just saying.

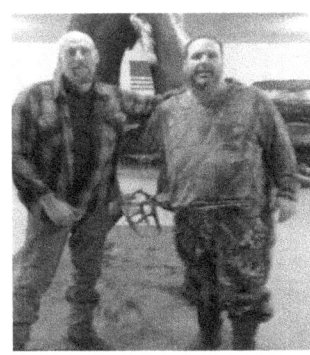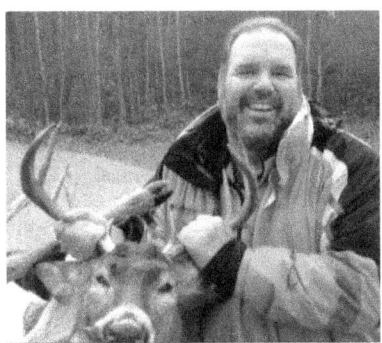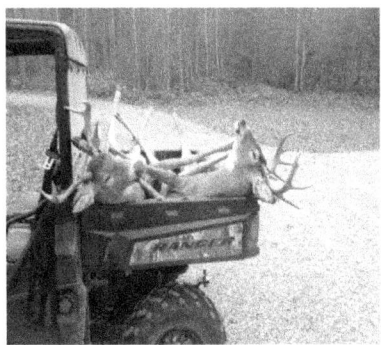

Gotta love the small town!! I must say, living in a small town has its advantages and disadvantages. One advantage is everyone seems to want to look out for you and the disadvantage is the same everyone is looking out for you. Case in point, many of the people in my little town know me personally. So many of them know about my health issues, up until I went to Vegas I didn't walk through town very often. So, you may have guessed it they are not used to seeing me walking the streets of town. It's kind of funny how many have stopped and asked me if I needed a ride somewhere. I usually just smile and say no just out for a stroll. One of these times I might revert to my smart-ass days and say "can you take me to the bank I need a getaway driver" or "maybe a lift to the asylum." Lol I am overdue for my evaluation. Don't get me wrong, it's nice that they car, but it is surprising that a fat guy out for a stroll is so newsworthy. I walked to town from deer camp yesterday, it was a three-mile one-way hike, needless to say out in the sticks where I was, there are not very many sidewalks. So, other than a couple of dirty looks from some of the drivers thinking that I was drunk already at noon walking down the side of the road. It wasn't such an event for the townspeople. For me though, it was a bucket list event. You see, I walked from camp to our favorite breakfast place and home which is a six-mile round trip. When I got there, I did have a bowl of chicken and vegetable soup, which I counted for my lunch. You might be getting to call B.S. bucket list event? Walking to a diner? I have been hunting with my buddy for 36 years, other than the second year I hunted at his new place and I spent the night in the woods, because I got lost and had to walk what seemed 100 miles to find his place. This was the longest scheduled excursion I have ever set out on foot for. Remember 108 days ago, I had about 15 feet of walking in me before I needed a rest. The other take away I got from the walk, was I only ordered the bowl of soup and a water. The dinner is known for their baked goods and you have to walk through the bakery to get to the restaurant. Dick move, I know right! But again, I feel myself exercising my will power muscle. Again, for you deer hunters out there, I am kinda ashamed to admit this one, but I have been in deer camo two days now and I have not had any alcohol. What's wrong with me!!! Lol

Pushing the envelope: We live in such a world of political correctness. Remember the part where we are always looking for government to police and protect us from ourselves. But in a time of our worst obesity statistics ever and a wave of healthy menu options out there, why would a restaurant chain target fat people the way this one does? I was going to disguise the name to protect the innocent, but then I figured they don't see the problem in it why should I. I guess they figure, since Wendy's used to use the slogan "where's the beef" and Burger King still uses "Home of the Whopper." Why shouldn't they be able to use Arby's "We have the meats." I guess I personally don't have a problem with that, but their latest advertising slogan leaves a little to be desired. Try our new pork belly sandwich. The first thing that comes to my deviant mind is a pork belly sandwich with a side of fat ass fries and a gallon of diet soda. Sounds like a cheeseburger away from a heart attack to me. They also make a sandwich, I should say a mountain of a sandwich that has 1.5 ounces of all of their meat, plus chicken tenders, plus cheese as well as your veggies and sauce. I am sure are well over 1000 calories sandwich only. Add curly fries and a cherry turnover and a diet soda of course and that's a healthy meal right there. Lol in their defense, they are not the only chain out there with extra-large menu choices, Burger King still sells a triple Whopper, McDonald's has their double quarter pounder with cheese. So, all the chains offer you the choices to be bad if you prefer. Remember no one is holding a gun to your head saying "eat fatty eat!!" Exercise that will power muscle and stay out of those situations where you have to choose between the temptations and chose to live instead.

Here is a list of the top 10 highest calorie fast food items.

FAST FOOD... OR JUST FAT FOOD? COUNTING THE CALORIES

1. White Castle - 20 chicken rings, **1,760 calories**

2. Burger King - Ultimate breakfast platter, **1,450 calories**

3. McDonald's - Big breakfast with syrup and margarine, **1,350 calories**

4. KFC - 10-piece bag of original recipe chicken bites, **1,300 calories**

5. Wendy's - Dave's Hot 'N Juicy 3/4 lb. triple patty with cheese, **1,120 calories**

6. Panera Bread - Steak and white cheddar on a French baguette, **980 calories**

7. Taco Bell - Volcanic nachos, **970 calories**

8. Dunkin' Donuts - Frozen mocha coffee coolatta with cream, **730 calories**

9. Subway - Mega melt on flatbread with egg, **660 calories**

10. Pizza Hut - 1 slice of a 14-inch large meat lover's pan pizza, **470 calories** Why stop there, since we like to push the envelope so much, here are some more sandwich only suggestions for you.

Triple Whopper with cheese

1230 calories

Double Quarter Pounder With Cheese

750 calories

Arby's - Meat Mountain

calories	1,275	Sodium	3,536 mg

Hardee's Megaburger

1,420 calories and 107 grams of fat.

Pick me! Pick Me! Pick Me! Do you remember when you were a kid, whenever you were getting ready to play a game. You would pick two captains, and they would choose two teams based on who was available to choose from. As a kid as well as an adult, you never wanted to be the last one chosen. So why do we always choose ourselves to be last in our daily lives? I know I get it, obligations!! As a spouse, we cater to the needs of our partner. As a parent, we cater to the needs of our kids. As an employee, we cater to the needs of our job. When do we ever cater to the needs of us? When we are dead ass tired or when we are sick, right? Exactly, that is what I am talking about. If you don't start making the right choices in your life starting with healthy food choices, the rest of it will be a moot point. What good are we to anyone but the doctor, when you are sick? The doctor and the pharmacy love seeing you, don't they? I can hear the cha Ching from here, even with my one good ear. Lol Seriously, the longer we put off taking care of ourselves, the worse we are going to get. Your body sends you signals, if we chose to ignore them, that is totally on us. After I have been thinking about this chapter, I don't think in my 51 years of existence hearing about anyone that was totally healthy, without any medical issues dropping dead for no apparent reason. I guess it could be possible, just highly unlikely.

Broaden your horizons: Ok so here is where honesty comes into play. So how many of you by show of hands, have not tried a food item because someone told you that it tastes like ass or even worse? No shaming here, it has happened to all of us at one point in our lives. No one wants to have an unfavorable taste left in their mouths. It's kinda like when someone asks you to try the milk, because it tastes spoiled to them and you try it anyway, just because the date on the outside says it should be ok, doesn't mean it still can't go bad. The lesson here, is that unless you try it, you would never know if you didn't like it. Do you have a friend that thinks they are allergic to everything they try? Now they may very well be, but highly unlikely. It might be the combination they are eating that may not be agreeing with their system, but you can't convince them of that, Right. For me it might be the name of the food item I can't get past. For me it is "cheese whiz" I guess I figure anything with the word "whiz" in it is kinda suspect. Most of my family likes it, I just haven't acquired a taste for it. Now that I try not to eat processed food, the chances of me adding it to my menu choices is pretty slim. A lot of us from our eating choices when we a young and never grow out of them or we are captive to what our parent ate and never broadened our flavor palette from there. Try not to get fixated on the name of the food, as much as how it tastes. For me I just started eating eggplant a lot. Eggplant is very good for you and it is one of the most versatile of vegetables. I guess you could call it the chameleon of vegetables because it takes on the flavor of whatever you cook it with. Another food that I have recently acquired a taste for is sweet potatoes, I don't know what stopped me from enjoying them at a younger age, but I love them now. Maybe it's the fact that since I have cut out sweets from my menu choices, I can substitute this health sweet option into my choices. The moral of the story is be your own person, try everything life has to offer, form your own opinions, and do what makes you feel the best. Just because you have never tried it or done it before, doesn't mean you will or won't like it. It's kinda like the ass comment, ass isn't for everyone, but some people like it. It doesn't make it wrong, it just makes it what it is.

Improvise, adapt, overcome: This has been one of my motto's ever since starting rehab. I think I may have heard it once in a marine movie or something. My therapist Beth used to accuse me of cheating. I would have to inform her that I was improvising and overcoming my obstacles, adapting to my environment, and excelling at my task at hand. She didn't like that response at the beginning of my treatments because it was different then she was accustomed to. Most people were not like me, they just did it the way she asked them to do it. Not me, this smart assed product of the sixties didn't play that game. Remember I was an overachiever that just had his life pretty much taken away during a 12-hour surgery. Therapy wasn't about baby steps; this was about getting stronger and remaining independent. I didn't have a choice to be lazy and let time heal everything. I was not a spring chicken and felt blessed to even get out of the hospital, much less continue to make progress. I have always been a problem solver; my brain never takes a holiday. I continue to look for the best ways to do things and hate, yes hate to do things this way because this is the way it has always been done. So, when it came to things I did before surgery and the way I had to do things after surgery I had a lot of adapting to do. Now add another fifty pounds or so onto an already weakened body. Bingo it sucked even more. I have to be honest, even being 100 pounds lighter it hasn't improved my balance at all. I definitely have more energy and stamina but I have not seen much residual improvement from the stroke symptoms. Does it mean I'm going to stop? Does it mean I'm going to give up? Hell, to the no, it just means that I am going to work even harder and change my stars to the outcome I decide, and not fall into being a statistic of what the establishment figures I would become after the stroke. On a side note, I gave one of my first drafts of this book to my therapist, because without all of her work challenging me. I know I wouldn't have been able to achieve the success I have seen so far. Thank you, Beth, and to the whole staff at The Tamerac Center for Wellness.

She loves me, she loves me not: This is a very difficult chapter to write, it is very personal, yet I felt it was important to the progress of my journey and there is a good chance you may encounter this situation as well. My wife and I have been through a lot over the 30 or so we have been together. Let's just say for me there have been more good than bad, but we have had our share of bad over the past eight years or so. I guess things started to head south in 2009 when my banking center closed after the economic downturn. SO, that triggered a slew of financial situations that required moving to another house, finding new employment, and a ton of new stress. Then add in the brain tumor in 2013 and the stroke at the end of 2013 and the long road back. Can you see where I am going with this. Oh, yes let's add in the fact that I lost two businesses during that time because I couldn't continue to take care of them and had to give up one of my greatest passions, coaching. I was pretty much in a tail spin. When you get married they don't give you an "if this happens, do this playbook." Right? They give you vows that kind of cover these situations. But not all situations I guess. So, I guess it is safe to say my wife and I have fallen out of love. I am not sure where this will lead to, but I am pretty sure it's not where I thought it was going to when we started our journey together on May, 28 1988. People grow apart, or lives take different paths, some things we control and some are out of our control. The key to so much of it is love and without it, you are just going through the motions. I thank God, every day that she stood by me through the surgery and stroke. It was her, my kids and family that gave me the strength to fight when it would have been so easy to give up. I guess maybe the changes in me after the surgery used up the last bit of love she had for me? She is still my best friend; we just lack the passion. I am not sure that it will ever come back, but I just wanted her to know she was the best thing that ever happened to me, besides my three kids. I know we had a bit of a spat when I was in Vegas around my birthday that affected my motivation to want to work out that day. It was at that point of my journey that I decided I couldn't let anyone not even my wife, derail me from my goal. Remember my goal is to get healthy. The weight loss is a byproduct of the journey. Getting healthy is a combination of body, mind, and soul. You need to get right with all three for the best chance to get healthy completely. I am no, Dr. Phil when it comes to these matters. I can only speak to my experience and all I know is that it has helped me continue on my journey. I know I will find love again. I have so much love to give and hopefully the healthier I get, the longer I will have to give it. On a personal note, for any skinny people still listening. Passion and sex are not the same thing, yes you can make love passionately but passion is also affection and kindness as well as the physical contact of even holding hands. You can sleep in the same bed only a foot away from each other and still feel miles away without the feel of a touch. I don't want to just sleep with someone, I want to wake up with someone I love and feel alive. Just saying.

Eating problem? I told you before I don't have an eating problem. I see food, I eat it, no problem. If it was only that easy to diagnose. Like I said before, everyone is different, yet they want to treat everyone the same when it comes to diet and nutrition. Unfortunately, this is not a one size fits all problem. Experimentation is the key I believe to what works for you. No I am not trying to discredit or downplay the qualifications of a dietician or medical professionals. But they don't know everything, and the makeup of everybody. This is why I keep harping on you to take ownership of your situation. Yes, you can take their advice, but you need to implement them in a way that helps you achieve your goals. Figure it out yourself, don't wait for someone else to tell you what's wrong with you. Listen to your body, rest it when it is tired, feed it when it is hungry. Give it nutrients and supplements to help it heal itself. But for God sake stop looking for someone to blame for the situation you are in. All that you are doing is wasting precious time you could be using to heal yourself. It doesn't matter how you got here or why you did, the only thing that matters is you get better. On the same note though, if you are living in a toxic situation or living with a fat person that seems to sabotage you whenever you start eating healthy, you may need to make a change to your residents before you can change your lifestyle. Just saying. I have a friend at the Tamerac that was in an abusive relationship for 21 years, she finally got up the courage to leave him, but before she left him she used his insurance to get bariatric surgery. She realized that the surgery wasn't going to cure all of her problems, but it was a start and the fact that his insurance had to pay for the surgery was a bonus for her.

Promises, promises, promises. I will start it tomorrow; I will work out tomorrow. I will listen to my body later, Is it tomorrow yet? I sure hope you make it to tomorrow, how about starting today? You ever hear the saying "no better, time than the present" or "why put off tomorrow, what you can do today?" I know they sound cliché, but so does waiting till it's too late, gets you dead. This is not a promise you are making to someone else, this is a promise you are making to you. You are not making a promise to your friend, or a customer or even your child. This is a promise that could affect the rest of your life. Remember, you are not cheating anyone but yourself, if you don't follow through with your promise this time. When you look at yourself in the mirror, are you able to say I did my best. Do I want to be here tomorrow, next week, next year or have I enjoyed as much has life had to offer me? If the answer is yes. God, bless you. If your answer is hell no, God bless you and great decision. Stop waiting for someone to give you permission to get healthy. Stop waiting for that magic pill that will make it easy. No one is saying it will be easy, but as you have figured out already, life is hard. Anything worth a damn, is worth working for. You are doing this for your very existence, isn't that reason enough? I hear it coming, B.S. aren't you being a little dramatic fat guy? No one has diagnosed me with anything yet! Exactly, that makes it even more important for you to start today. Why wait until you get sentenced to something? Be proactive and keep the bad news from ever reaching you, or not, a lifetime of medication for high blood pressure, or sticking yourself daily checking your blood sugar or even injections daily of insulin, is a much better solution. Life is about choices, choose LIFE!!

If you ain't cheating, you ain't trying! Ever hear the saying "if you ain't cheating, you ain't trying?" It kinda ties in with a couple of rants I have thrown at you. I guess I need to clarify what cheating is to me. Cheating to me is adapting to the best way I can do something, no it doesn't mean doing things half-assed, or cutting work outs short or even skipping workouts and saying I did them. Remember you are not cheating anyone but yourself here. There is no trophy waiting here for the winner, no banquet at the end of the journey and we sure the hell are not going for ice cream when it is over either. So, you can get that right out of your sick mind right quick now. In this rant cheating means you are doing everything you can do, that you can do your way. I hope that makes sense. All of us have limitations, most exercises are invented with healthy athletic people in mind to perform them. Now that we have exceeded the limits of their expectation, we still can find benefit from doing their exercise routines. With modifications, of course. I don't know about you, but as of 108 days ago, I had trouble seeing my feet, much less touching them. I still have problems today with that, but at least it is possible. One of my biggest ah ha moments so far when it comes to my body is how tight your muscles get when you don't use them, for any length of time or if you use them in a limited capacity. Because of my balance issues, I walked with old man syndrome, old man syndrome is where you take very short strides and shuffle your feet. I did that out of fear of falling, but as a result the tendons in my legs got really tight and don't have very much mobility. I started walking backwards and side to side in the pool and that has helped loosen them up. They are not perfect yet but on the road to recovery. I ranted before about the Nutrisystem claim to have chemical that will target belly fat, I have no problem calling B.S. on that one. The only thing I know that targets belly fat is sit ups and ab crunches which for me were not a good option. I did start doing them in the pool holding onto the pool ladder. I have to say I have seen an improvement in my mid-section. Am I getting the same benefit doing them in the pool as if I did them on land? I guess I would have to answer that with another question. If I don't do them on land because I find them to be painful or too strenuous, is that cheating? Just saying.

Less is more!! Have you ever heard anyone say this little gem to you? It's kinda like when someone says "Same difference?" how can something be the same and different at the same time? But for this rant, it will make sense, trust me. So, last week I spent the second half of the week in the woods remember. "Hunting" right? Other than walking all over God's Country and loading and unloading sugar beets, that was about it on the exercise front. I did focus a great deal on what I put in my mouth though. I was pretty concerned when it came to weigh ins this week. Not so much for me if it was only me, but I have a teammate for this challenge and I didn't want to let her down. So officially I lost five pounds this week. I was pretty ecstatic, No, it wasn't the eight I was shooting for, but I did realize that my body carries four pounds of water weight on a daily basis. It seems that if I weigh myself after my workouts, I am always four pounds less. So, I lost nine pounds last week if I subtract my water weight. I like that number better. My book, my number lol This is a great time to reiterate my hate, yes hate for scales, weight, and weight loss. To me all that does is keeps me living in a skinny person's world. I would rather be judged on how I feel and right now, I am feeling pretty damn good. My flexibility is up; my stamina is up and my motivation level is up as well. The fact that my weight keeps dropping is a bonus.

Don't judge a book by its cover!! You bought this book still didn't you and thank you very much by the way. This rant has to do with judging people, you don't know their story and even if you know their story, unless you are them you only know half of the story at best. I my bitch about people in this book about times when they get in the way of my workouts. But I never try to downplay or minimalize their efforts and their workout routines. Case in point, I have not seen a woman for a little over a week in the pool. I actually wrote a little rant about her earlier in the book. Not so much about her specifically, but what I perceived as a useless workout. If you have a better memory than I do, it was the rant about people that just float in the pool and wiggle their toes and consider that a work out. This is the reason I try my hardest not to judge. So not seeing her again today in the pool, I asked one of the other regulars, if they knew where she has been? They informed me that she lost her battle with cancer. See she like as I shared the freedom and comfort of the pool to feel free from the strain gravity puts on our bodies and mobility. She liked to float in the pool and swim her cares away. I can totally relate to that feeling. I wish her Godspeed on the completion of her journey and may she resonate with us as the reason not to judge others. So I had an AH HA moment today. I am visiting my daughter Andrea, in Virginia Beach. I am here without a car; her place is close to most everything. So, I decided to walk to the store to get some groceries. As I was waiting at the corner of the busy intersection carrying my snazzy new Trader Joe's colorful bag of groceries. I couldn't help to think what all the cars were thinking as they whizzed by. "Look at the fat guy carrying the bags of groceries, maybe if he didn't eat so much he could afford a car." Came to mind more than once. Then I thought to myself, self they don't know me. They don't know that I have five cars registered in my name right now. They don't know that I walked 12 miles yesterday as exercise. God forgive them for they do not know! Moral of the story is, we will all atone for our thoughts and sins at one point in our lives. The more times we don't pass judgement on people we don't know, the less we will have to atone for when it's our time to be judged. Just Saying.

So, you're ready for your first three way, Ay? Ok down fat guys, put the lil chubby's away. So, you have decided to take the challenge and start your own journey. Yes, it can feel scary going out on your own. Remember there is safety in numbers. Have you ever heard the saying, "me, myself and I?" I know it's been awhile since I had a math class, but that would be three in my book. Ok, fat guy, cute but there is still only one of me standing here. You are so correct, but at our size we are two to three of a skinny person, am I, right? I am asking you to stretch and think out of the box here. I am a firm believer, that our body has three key ingredients to success and good health. The body, mind, and soul. To break it down even more the brain, heart, and body. In my opinion you cannot LIVE without any one of them. Notice I didn't say stay alive. They have ways to keep us alive even though we are not living our lives. The journey can be a lonely one, especially if you don't use your imagination. No I am not saying carry on a conversation with yourself. But my mother always said, there is nothing wrong with talking to yourself, the problem comes in when you start answering. Lol The biggest thing to remember is yes, this is your journey. What are you doing it for, why are you doing it? Share that information with yourself. I know that may sound silly, but you would be surprised the games fat people play even against themselves. For example, I told you earlier I was on my journey to hopefully earn more years to spend with my family. My body wasn't always in the mood to work out eight hours a day. That is when my brain and heart would team up against it and help me recall a memory of maybe my wedding day or when one of my children were born and I would remember why I was doing this, and the it helped me get through that day. There were some days when my heart wasn't feeling it and my brain and body, worked together to prepare a healthy meal that day. It might have even been a meal that would strike a chord with one of my heart strings and tie all three units back together. So never think that you are alone in this fight. Share the fight with your entire body. You are all in it together anyway. Just so the fat guys don't want to jump me after they get done reading this rant, thinking that I am a tease. Then Trixie and her twin sister Pixie put their clothes back on and made a fruit smoothie and went home for the night... Better?

Trick or treat? No, no and hell no!! Just to get that out of the way. This is not a game, there is no room in this journey for failure. Tricks are not the way to win trust with your body, honesty is. Time to go through the house and throw away your secret stash's also. It's not an out of sight, out of mind game. Yes, if you hide it in the house, the temptation is going to drive you out of your mind. This is where your loved one's support is going to be tested. No, they are not on this journey with you. They should be able to enjoy their guilty pleasures, if they want to, I get that. But on the same token, it shouldn't be enjoyed in front of you and it shouldn't be left for you to be tempted with after they are done with it either. This is why I say family make horrible support groups. They are willing to help you, but generally not at the expense of changing their regiment and I guess if they are fit and healthy, it must be working for them, right? Even if they are dumping unhealthy food down their throats is that the best thing for them to do either? Just because they weigh less than you, does it make it, right? So, I just returned home from a four-day hunting trip, with my best friend. First, I have to say it was the weirdest deer camp we have had in the 36 years we have been hunting together. It started out weird, based on all the healthy food I prepped and took with me. Second, it was the first time since we became legal to drink alcohol, that I didn't consume one, at deer camp or the tavern we went to. Third other than walking and loading sugar beets, that was the only exercise I did all weekend. Forth, we ate some great food this weekend, so it's not like it was all salads and water. Fifth, I was a bit scared to get on the scale today and before I worked out I lost seven pounds from last week. To say I was ecstatic, was an understatement. Probably the highlight of the weekend though, was the fact that my buddy read a draft of the book and understood not only why I did what I did, but implemented some of my changes into how he prepared the meals also. Last but certainly not least, I crossed off another bucket list item and lived long enough to experience another deer camp with my best friend. 109 days ago, I had to put it on the list of things I hoped I would be able to do again and all the hard work so far bought me one more camp, to date. So, I feel the need to scream bull shit on this little gem too. Parents that drag their infants around for miles just so they can score tons of unneeded candy and treats. Give me a break, nothing pisses me of more than having some parent push their something month old baby up to my candy stand, and the kid can't even speak yet say trick or treat but the parent has no problem holding their plastic pumpkin out to get candy that this child was no business even having in their stroller, much less anything else with it. I have even had pregnant mothers come up and ask for candy for the one on the way, tell me that's not bull shit. Remember one of the first steps to recovery is admitting you have a problem. If you are using your infant child to score some free candy, you are a redneck but you also have a sugar problem. Just saying

Pretty little secrets, pretty little lies: I think it was Don Henley that sang the song "Dirty Laundry." We all have some as well as guilty pleasures. I just mentioned going to deer camp with my best friend of 48 years. He still hides the fact that he smokes from me. He has been doing it for years. He is also 52 years old, I don't know what he is so worried about me finding out for. We have done some crazy things in our past, smoking is pretty low on the list. Secrets are a slippery slope though. The guilt people feel from keeping secrets along with the added stress from keeping the secrets from our loved ones, leads to unhealthy lifestyle situations. You hear all the time about stress eaters or stress drinkers. I know coming clean is a very hard thing to do and again I am not Dr. Phil but I know for me at least, coming clean with as many of my demons as possible has allowed me to continue on my journey and continue my success. One of the biggest traps we fall into in weight loss programs is not setting goals and expectations. We just expect the weight to continue to fall off on its own. I know personally I am not satisfied with losing anything less than eight lbs. a week. Yes, I know that is unrealistic, but it is something to shoot for. If I shoot for eight and I hit six, it's not horrible, right? On the same token if I aim for eight and hit 10, then bonus right. You might be thinking where the fat guy picked the number eight from? There are seven days in a week, I expect to lose a pound a day so that's seven, right? Then I consider myself an over achiever so that's where the eighth pound comes from. That's all fine and good, but you need to have a plan when you shoot for eight and hit two or even worse, gain weight. Then what? That's where the journals come in handy, look back at what you did last week, did you do all you could do exercise wise? Did you forget to list something that you ate??? Remember you're not cheating anyone but yourself here, this is a pretty high stakes game you are playing. Can you afford to lose? If you go through the journal and it all checks out and you still gained, then you have to make adjustments to your regiment. Ladies here is one of God's cruel jokes I recently found out from my challenge partner. Last week she was doing great at the beginning of the week, then Aunt Flow came a calling and she retained water the second half of the week. She ended up even for the week, but I felt horrible for her. Besides dealing with all the B.S. associated with the menstrual cycle, she still battled to keep from gaining weight. Great job Cass.

Food is a horrible drug!!!

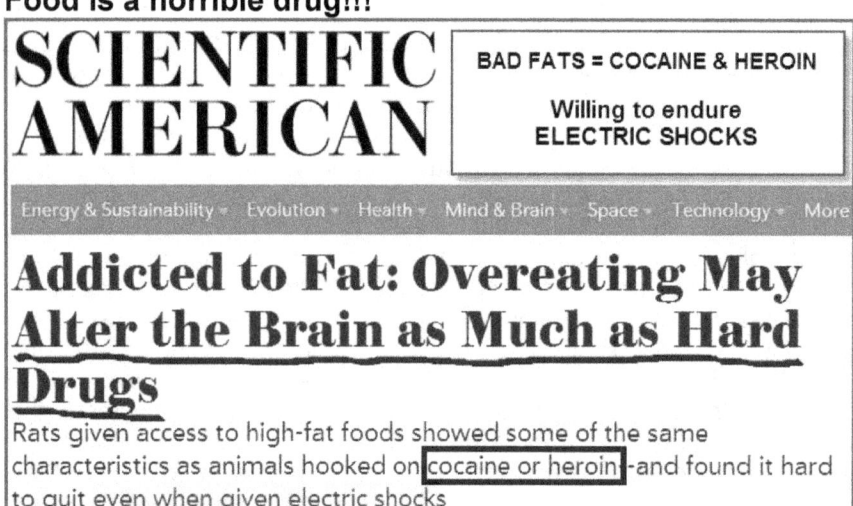

I am sure this next rant is going to strike a nerve for many of the establishment type folks out there as well as people in the medical world, but again this is weight loss through the eyes of this fat guy. Thank God, I live in a country where the freedom of speech is still protected. Rant locked and loaded sir!! You thought Big Pharm. Was our biggest problem, how can we see the forest through the trees when it comes to our food choices? No I don't mean healthy food choices, or do I? We live in the greatest country on earth, Yes, I know it is debatable sometimes, but for this fat guy, there is no place I would rather be then the U.S. of A. We live in the world of free enterprise and with that brings the endless supply of choices. Really how many variety of candy bars do we actually need and why are they always located in a place where you are bored out of your mind waiting in line to check out and can't wait to get to your car and rip open your box of Twinkies? Can I get a high five!! So instead you rationalize the nutritional value between the king-sized snickers staring you in the hairy eyeball, or the Twinkie that has an endless shelf life, but is likewise delish!! Then you make the adult like executive decision, I will choose the king-sized Snicker bar because it won't hurt to put the Twinkie's on the shelf for the one or two days depending how many mouths you have in your household to consume that box and I will eat my precious in the car or at the checkout as soon as I feel safe that my debit card isn't going to be declined. Don't lie to me fat people, we have all been there. Talking about the debit card decline. No one would ever rationalize the choice between a Snickers and a Twinkie, they are two different food groups, right? Snickers is a candy and a Twinkie is a bread so it's all good, look it up on that pyramid thingy I am sure they taught us that back in school somewhere. I know that's the lighter side to the real problem facing fat people today, so many choices so little time. Obesity is a national epidemic; it leads to more deaths than every other cause of death known to mankind. Wait a minute fat guy do you have proof of that. No, remember I am just a fat guy spewing my rants, but remember I do have a history of being fat and even though I only hear out of one ear now since the surgery God has still blessed me with two eyes and the ability to hear pretty damned good out of my right ear. Obesity is one of the main causes for the following according to the National Heart, Lung, and Blood Institute.

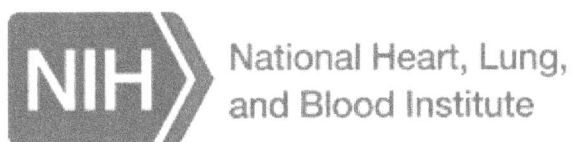
National Heart, Lung,
and Blood Institute

What Are the Health Risks of Overweight and Obesity?

Being overweight or obese isn't a cosmetic problem. These conditions greatly raise your risk for other health problems.

Overweight and Obesity-Related Health Problems in Adults

Coronary Heart Disease

As your body mass index rises, so does your risk for coronary heart disease (CHD). CHD is a condition in which a waxy substance called plaque (plak) builds up inside the coronary arteries. These arteries supply oxygen-rich blood to your heart.
Plaque can narrow or block the coronary arteries and reduce blood flow to the heart muscle. This can cause angina (an-JI-nuh or AN-juh-nuh) or a heart attack. (Angina is chest pain or discomfort.)
Obesity also can lead to heart failure. This is a serious condition in which your heart can't pump enough blood to meet your body's needs.

High Blood Pressure

Blood pressure is the force of blood pushing against the walls of the arteries as the heart pumps blood. If this pressure rises and stays high over time, it can damage the body in many ways.
Your chances of having high blood pressure are greater if you're overweight or obese.

Stroke

Being overweight or obese can lead to a buildup of plaque in your arteries. Eventually, an area of plaque can rupture, causing a blood clot to form.
If the clot is close to your brain, it can block the flow of blood and oxygen to your brain and cause a stroke. The risk of having a stroke rises as BMI increases.

Type 2 Diabetes

Diabetes is a disease in which the body's blood glucose, or blood sugar, level is too high. Normally, the body breaks down food into glucose and then carries it to cells throughout the body. The cells use a hormone called insulin to turn the glucose into energy.
In type 2 diabetes, the body's cells don't use insulin properly. At first, the body reacts by making more insulin. Over time, however, the body can't make enough insulin to control its blood sugar level.
Diabetes is a leading cause of early death, CHD, stroke, kidney disease, and blindness. Most people who have type 2 diabetes are overweight.

Abnormal Blood Fats

If you're overweight or obese, you're at increased risk of having abnormal levels of blood fats. These include high levels of triglycerides and LDL ("bad") cholesterol and low levels of HDL ("good") cholesterol.
Abnormal levels of these blood fats are a risk factor for CHD. For more information about triglycerides and LDL and HDL cholesterol, go to the Health Topics High Blood Cholesterol article.
Metabolic syndrome is the name for a group of risk factors that raises your risk for heart disease and other health problems, such as diabetes and stroke.
You can develop any one of these risk factors by itself, but they tend to occur together. A diagnosis of metabolic syndrome is made if you have at least three of the following risk factors:

- A large waistline. This is called abdominal obesity or "having an apple shape." Having extra fat in the waist area is a greater risk factor for CHD than having extra fat in other parts of the body, such as on the hips.
- A higher than normal triglyceride level (or you're on medicine to treat high triglycerides).
- A lower than normal HDL cholesterol level (or you're on medicine to treat low HDL cholesterol).

- Higher than normal blood pressure (or you're on medicine to treat high blood pressure).

- Higher than normal fasting blood sugar (or you're on medicine to treat diabetes).

Cancer

Being overweight or obese raises your risk for colon, breast, endometrial, and gallbladder cancers. Osteoarthritis is a common joint problem of the knees, hips, and lower back. The condition occurs if the tissue that protects the joints wears away. Extra weight can put more pressure and wear on joints, causing pain.

Sleep apnea is a common disorder in which you have one or more pauses in breathing or shallow breaths while you sleep.

A person who has sleep apnea may have more fat stored around the neck. This can narrow the airway, making it hard to breathe.

Obesity hypoventilation syndrome (OHS) is a breathing disorder that affects some obese people. In OHS, poor breathing results in too much carbon dioxide (hypoventilation) and too little oxygen in the blood (hypoxemia).

OHS can lead to serious health problems and may even cause death

Reproductive Problems

Obesity can cause menstrual issues and infertility in women.

Gallstones

Gallstones are hard pieces of stone-like material that form in the gallbladder. They're mostly made of cholesterol. Gallstones can cause stomach or back pain.

People who are overweight or obese are at increased risk of having gallstones. Also, being overweight may result in an enlarged gallbladder that doesn't work well.

Overweight and Obesity-Related Health Problems in Children and Teens

Overweight and obesity also increase the health risks for children and teens. Type 2 diabetes once was rare in American children, but an increasing number of children are developing the disease.

Also, overweight children are more likely to become overweight or obese as adults, with the same disease risks.

So, if obesity is one of the main causes of heart disease, stroke, cancer, hypertension, diabetes and so on and so on. How could it not be considered a pandemic colossal reason to help control fat people syndrome? Easy, food is not an illegal substance. Everything out of moderation has the potential to kill you, should we put a ban on everything? The FDA's job is to regulate what a manufacturer puts on a label is actually what it is. They also try to monitor that food is kept free of poisons and are stored at the proper temperatures so we don't die of an immediate death, but remember the goal of any business is to not kill its customers quickly right. If they get 20 or 30 years of your money they win, right? So, what are you saying fat guy? Big brother needs more regulations to save us from ourselves? No wise ass, I am saying we need to start saving ourselves from ourselves. I will be one of the first to scream B.S. if anyone wants to blame the government for us being fat. All I want from the government is to make sure the manufacturers post the correct information on the packaging. Stop allowing them to slick talk us into thinking that it's ok to eat a million-calorie product without knowing how bad it really is for us. Didn't they do that with the cigarette companies and look how much that did for us? I agree a warning label of the side of a snickers bar is not the answer, remember most fat people don't read past the giant SNICKERS on the front of the candy bar. The only way I see the situation of obesity to get better is keep your mouth shut. No I don't mean stop talking about the problem, I mean stop eating the problem. Start focusing on eating healthy and leave the empty or bad calorie foods on the shelf. That doesn't mean that you go back in a couple of weeks and buy them at a discount because they have marked them down because their expiration date is fast approaching, remember a Twinkie has like a 50-year shelf life. I am saying treat everything like a Twinkie, put all the crap on proverbial shelf and don't touch it for 50 years, if you still want it 50 years from now, God willing we are still on this planet then eat away. Just saying the choice is yours

How to Understand and Use the Nutrition Facts Label

U.S. Department of Health and Human Services
NOTE: FDA has issued final changes to update the Nutrition Facts label for packaged foods. For more information, see.

People look at food labels for different reasons. But whatever the reason, many consumers would like to know how to use this information more effectively and easily. The following label-building skills are intended to make it easier for you to use nutrition labels to make quick, informed food choices that contribute to a healthy diet.

The information in the main or top section (see #1-4 and #6 on the sample nutrition label below), can vary with each food product; it contains product-specific information (serving size, calories, and nutrient information). The bottom part (see #5 on the sample label below) contains a footnote with Daily Values (DVs) for 2,000 and 2,500 calorie diets. This footnote provides recommended dietary information for important nutrients, including fats, sodium, and fiber. The footnote is found only on larger packages and does not change from product to product.

In the following Nutrition Facts label we have colored certain sections to help you focus on those areas that will be explained in detail. You will not see these colors on the food labels on products you purchase.
Sample Label for Macaroni and Cheese

1. The Serving Size

(#1 on sample label)
The first place to start when you look at the Nutrition Facts label is the serving size and the number of servings in the package. Serving sizes are standardized to make it easier to compare similar foods; they are provided in familiar units, such as cups or pieces, followed by the metric amount, e.g., the number of grams.

The size of the serving on the food package influences the number of calories and all the nutrient amounts listed on the top part of the label. Pay attention to the serving size, especially how many servings there are in the food package. Then ask yourself, "How many servings am I consuming"? (e.g., 1/2 serving, 1 serving, or more) In the sample label, one serving of macaroni and cheese equals one cup. If you ate the whole package, you would eat two cups. That doubles the calories and other nutrient numbers, including the %Daily Values as shown in the sample label.

Example				
	Single Serving	%DV	Double Serving	%DV
Serving Size	1 cup (228g)		2 cups (456g)	
Calories	250		500	
Calories from Fat	110		220	
Total Fat	12g	18%	24g	36%
Trans Fat	1.5g		3g	
Saturated Fat	3g	15%	6g	30%
Cholesterol	30mg	10%	60mg	20%
Sodium	470mg	20%	940mg	40%
Total Carbohydrate	31g	10%	62g	20%
Dietary Fiber	0g	0%	0g	0%

Sugars	5g		10g	
Protein	5g		10g	
Vitamin A		4%		8%
Vitamin C		2%		4%
Calcium		20%		40%
Iron		4%		8%

2. Calories (and Calories from Fat)

Calories provide a measure of how much energy you get from a serving of this food. Many Americans consume more calories than they need without meeting recommended intakes for a number of nutrients. The calorie section of the label can help you manage your weight (i.e., gain, lose, or maintain.)
Remember: the number of servings you consume determines the number of calories you eat (your portion amount).
(#2 on sample label)
In the example, there are 250 calories in one serving of this macaroni and cheese. How many calories from fat are there in ONE serving? Answer: 110 calories, which means almost half the calories in a single serving come from fat. What if you ate the whole package content? Then, you would consume two servings, or 500 calories, and 220 would come from fat.
General Guide to Calories
· 40 Calories is low
· 100 Calories is moderate
· 400 Calories or more is high
The General Guide to Calories provides a general reference for calories when you look at a Nutrition Facts label. This guide is based on a 2,000-calorie diet.
Eating too many calories per day is linked to overweight and obesity.

3 and 4. The Nutrients: How Much?

Look at the top of the nutrient section in the sample label. It shows you some key nutrients that impact on your health and separates them into two main groups:

Limit These Nutrients

(#3 on sample label)
The nutrients listed first are the ones Americans generally eat in adequate amounts, or even too much. They are identified in yellow as Limit these Nutrients. Eating too much fat, saturated fat, *trans* fat, cholesterol, or sodium may increase your risk of certain chronic diseases, like heart disease, some cancers, or high blood pressure.
Important: Health experts recommend that you keep your intake of saturated fat, *trans* fat and cholesterol as low as possible as part of a nutritionally balanced diet.

Get Enough of These

(#4 on sample label)
Most Americans don't get enough dietary fiber, vitamin A, vitamin C, calcium, and iron in their diets. They are identified in blue as Get Enough of these Nutrients. Eating enough of these nutrients can improve your health and help reduce the risk of some diseases and conditions. For example, getting enough calcium may reduce the risk of osteoporosis, a condition that results in brittle bones as one ages (see calcium section below). Eating a diet high in dietary fiber promotes healthy bowel function. Additionally, a diet rich in fruits, vegetables, and grain products that contain dietary fiber, particularly soluble fiber, and low in saturated fat and cholesterol may reduce the risk of heart disease.
Remember: You can use the Nutrition Facts label not only to help *limit* those nutrients you want to cut back on but also to *increase* those nutrients you need to consume in greater amounts.

5. Understanding the Footnote on the Bottom of the Nutrition Facts Label
(#5 on sample label)

Note the * used after the heading "%Daily Value" on the Nutrition Facts label. It refers to the Footnote in the lower part of the nutrition label, which tells you "%DVs are based on a 2,000-calorie diet". This statement must be on all food labels. But the remaining information in the full footnote may not be on the package if the size of the label is too small. When the full footnote does appear, it will always be the same. It doesn't change from product to product, because it shows recommended dietary advice for all Americans--it is not about a specific food product.

Look at the amounts circled in red in the footnote--these are the Daily Values (DV) for each nutrient listed and are based on public health experts' advice. DVs are recommended levels of intakes. DVs in the footnote are based on a 2,000 or 2,500 calorie diet. Note how the DVs for some nutrients change, while others (for cholesterol and sodium) remain the same for both calorie amounts.

How the Daily Values Relate to the %DVs

Look at the example below for another way to see how the Daily Values (DVs) relate to the %DVs and dietary guidance. For each nutrient listed there is a DV, a %DV, and dietary advice or a goal. If you follow this dietary advice, you will stay within public health experts recommended upper or lower limits for the nutrients listed, based on a 2,000-calorie daily diet.

Examples of DVs versus %DVs

Based on a 2,000 Calorie Diet

Nutrient	DV	%DV	Goal
Total Fat	65g	= 100%DV	Less than
Sat Fat	20g	= 100%DV	Less than
Cholesterol	300mg	= 100%DV	Less than
Sodium	2400mg	= 100%DV	Less than
Total Carbohydrate	300g	= 100%DV	At least
Dietary Fiber	25g	= 100%DV	At least

Upper Limit - Eat "Less than"...

The nutrients that have "upper daily limits" are listed first on the footnote of larger labels and on the example, above. Upper limits means it is recommended that you stay below - eat "less than" - the Daily Value nutrient amounts listed per day. For example, the DV for Saturated fat (in the yellow section) is 20g. This amount is 100% DV for this nutrient. What is the goal or dietary advice? To eat "less than" 20 g or 100%DV for the day.<

Lower Limit - Eat "At least"...

Now look at the section in blue where dietary fiber is listed. The DV for dietary fiber is 25g, which is 100% DV. This means it is recommended that you eat "at least" this amount of dietary fiber per day.

The DV for Total Carbohydrate (section in white) is 300g or 100%DV. This amount is recommended for a balanced daily diet that is based on 2,000 calories, but can vary, depending on your daily intake of fat and protein.

Now let's look at the %DVs.

6. The Percent Daily Value (%DV)

The % Daily Values (%DVs) are based on the Daily Value recommendations for key nutrients but only for a 2,000-calorie daily diet--not 2,500 calories. You, like most people, may not know how many calories you consume in a day. But you can still use the %DV as a frame of reference whether or not you consume more or less than 2,000 calories.

The %DV helps you determine if a serving of food is high or low in a nutrient. Note: a few nutrients, like *trans*-fat, do not have a %DV--they will be discussed later.

Do you need to know how to calculate percentages to use the %DV? No, the label (the %DV) does the math for you. It helps you interpret the numbers (grams and milligrams) by putting them all on the same scale for the day (0-100%DV). The %DV column doesn't add up vertically to 100%. Instead each nutrient is based on 100% of the daily requirements for that nutrient (for a 2,000-calorie diet). This way you can tell high from low and know which nutrients contribute a lot, or a little, to your daily recommended allowance (upper or lower).

Quick Guide to %DV

5%DV or less is low and 20%DV or more is high
(#6 on sample label)
This guide tells you that 5%DV or less is low for all nutrients, those you want to limit (e.g., fat, saturated fat, cholesterol, and sodium), or for those that you want to consume in greater amounts (fiber, calcium, etc.). As the Quick Guide shows, 20%DV or more is high for all nutrients.
Example: Look at the amount of Total Fat in one serving listed on the sample nutrition label. Is 18%DV contributing a lot or a little to your fat limit of 100% DV? Check the Quick Guide to %DV. 18%DV, which is below 20%DV, is not yet high, but what if you ate the whole package (two servings)? You would double that amount, eating 36% of your daily allowance for Total Fat. Coming from just one food, that amount leaves you with 64% of your fat allowance (100%-36%=64%) for *all* of the other foods you eat that day, snacks and drinks included.

| 1 serving |
| 2 servings |

Using the %DV

Comparisons: The %DV also makes it easy for you to make comparisons. You can compare one product or brand to a similar product. Just make sure the serving sizes are similar, especially the weight (e.g. gram, milligram, ounces) of each product. It's easy to see which foods are higher or lower in nutrients because the serving sizes are generally consistent for similar types of foods, (see the comparison example at the end) except in a few cases like cereals.
Nutrient Content Claims: Use the %DV to help you quickly distinguish one claim from another, such as "reduced fat" vs. "light" or "nonfat." Just compare the %DVs for Total Fat in each food product to see which one is higher or lower in that nutrient--there is no need to memorize definitions. This works when comparing all nutrient content claims, e.g., less, light, low, free, more, high, etc.
Dietary Trade-Offs: You can use the %DV to help you make dietary trade-offs with other foods throughout the day. You don't have to give up a favorite food to eat a healthy diet. When a food you like is high in fat, balance it with foods that are low in fat at other times of the day. Also, pay attention to how much you eat so that the total amount of fat for the day stays below 100%DV.

Nutrients With a %DV but No Weight Listed - Spotlight on Calcium

Calcium: Look at the %DV for calcium on food packages so you know how much one serving contributes to the *total amount you need* per day. Remember, a food with 20%DV or more contributes a lot of calcium to your daily total, while one with 5%DV or less contributes a little.

Experts advise adult consumers to consume adequate amounts of calcium, that is, 1,000mg or 100%DV in a daily 2,000 calorie diet. This advice is often given in milligrams (mg), but the Nutrition Facts label only lists a %DV for calcium.

For food skim

Equivalencies
30% DV = 300mg calcium = one cup of milk
100% DV = 1,000mg calcium
130% DV = 1,300mg calcium

certain populations, they advise that adolescents, especially girls, consume 1,300mg (130%DV) and post-menopausal women consume 1,200mg (120%DV) of calcium daily. The DV for calcium on labels is 1,000mg.

Don't be fooled -- always check the label for calcium because you can't make assumptions about the amount of calcium in specific food categories. Example: the amount of calcium in milk, whether or whole, is generally the same per serving, whereas the amount of calcium in the same size yogurt container (8oz) can vary from 20-45 %DV.

Nutrients Without a %DV: *Trans* Fats, Protein, and Sugars:

Note that *Trans*-fat, Sugars and, Protein do not list a %DV on the Nutrition Facts label.

Plain Yogurt

Fruit Yogurt

Trans Fat: Experts could not provide a reference value for *trans*-fat nor any other information that FDA believes is sufficient to establish a Daily Value or %DV. Scientific reports link *trans*-fat (and saturated fat) with raising blood LDL ("bad") cholesterol levels, both of which increase your risk of coronary heart disease, a leading cause of death in the US.

Important: Health experts recommend that you keep your intake of saturated fat, *trans* fat and cholesterol as low as possible as part of a nutritionally balanced diet.

Protein: A %DV is required to be listed if a claim is made for protein, such as "high in protein". Otherwise, unless the food is meant for use by infants and children under 4 years old, none is needed. Current scientific evidence indicates that protein intake is not a public health concern for adults and children over 4 years of age.

Sugars: No daily reference value has been established for sugars because no recommendations have been made for the total amount to eat in a day. Keep in mind, the sugars listed on the Nutrition Facts label include naturally occurring sugars (like those in fruit and milk) as well as those added to a food or drink. Check the ingredient list for specifics on added sugars.

Take a look at the Nutrition Facts label for the two yogurt examples. The plain yogurt on the left has 10g of sugars, while the fruit yogurt on the right has 44g of sugars in one serving.

Now look below at the ingredient lists for the two yogurts. Ingredients are listed in descending order of weight (from most to least). Note that no added sugars or sweeteners are in the list of ingredients for the plain yogurt, yet 10g of sugars were listed on the Nutrition Facts label. This is because there are no added sugars in plain yogurt, only naturally occurring sugars (lactose in the milk).

Plain Yogurt - contains no added sugars

Fruit Yogurt - contains added sugars

If you are concerned about your intake of sugars, make sure that added sugars are not listed as one of the first few ingredients. Other names for added sugars include: corn syrup, high-fructose corn syrup, fruit juice concentrate, maltose, dextrose, sucrose, honey, and maple syrup.

To limit nutrients that have no %DV, like *trans*-fat and sugars, compare the labels of similar products and choose the food with the lowest amount.

Comparison Example

Below are two kinds of milk- one is "Reduced Fat," the other is "Nonfat" milk. Each serving size is one cup. Which has more calories and more saturated fat? Which one has more calcium?

REDUCED FAT MILK - 2% Milkfat	NONFAT MILK

Answer: As you can see, they both have the same amount of calcium, but the nonfat milk has no saturated fat and has 40 calories less per serving than the reduced fat milk.

FDA
U.S. Food and Drug Administration
10903 New Hampshire Avenue
Silver Spring, MD 20993
1-888-INFO-FDA (1-888-463-6332)

Ok, so now that we know how to read the label, now what? Do it! Know what you are putting in your body. Challenge yourself to eliminate empty calories, preservatives, chemicals. If they don't make a natural substitute, then you need to ask yourself, should I be putting this in my body? I know I know, I hear the bull shits from a mile away, but fat guy, it's so easy for you, "you know how to cook." We must eat all this processed crap, that is frozen or ready to eat! And I call bull shit right back on you!! Learn, if you don't know how to do something learn! The cooking channel, internet, hell open a book! It might not be Martha Stewart worthy your first try, but what doesn't kill you makes you stronger right? All I am saying is, you get one body and one lifetime, protect it, take care of it and it will take care of you. Don't and you're in for a world of hurt. Just Saying.
High Fructose Corn Syrup: Better known as HFCS or Poison by some.
So why do I say that? Fat guy, it's made from corn, what's the problem? So, is ethanol, you don't see me putting gas on my Fruit Loops, do you? Here is a fat camp challenge for you. Next time you are at the grocery store, try to find five things that don't contain high fructose corn syrup in them. Good luck! Let me give you some facts, while you are on your quest.
Now, remember, I am not a doctor or any other professional and these are just pictures. I don't have any scientific proof that back these claims up. But considering I have had at least half of these side effects listed above. Coincidence? I think not. Have you found your five items yet? I doubt that too. It will take you a good bit of time to do that. The biggest reason companies went away from using regular sugar, was cost. They went to this chemically modified product, because it is cheaper. Cheaper is better, Right?

So here is a little information I just picked up on where the hell the FDA came up with the 2000 calorie's a day formula posted on the back of everything we eat. If you can figure it out, you are smarter than me. This is why I say " listen to your body."

Why 2000 Calories?

When developing the new food label, the Food and Drug Administration needed a base for % Daily Values — a new feature to help customers see at a glance the fat and other nutrient content of a certain food. A mathematically simple 2,000 calorie-a-day diet was chosen so that consumers could easily calculate the Daily Values needed for their own diets.

This is the amount of total calories per day that a moderately active adult female (weighing approximately 132 pounds) would need to maintain her weight. However, if you do not fit this description, your caloric needs will vary. It is important, therefore, that you adapt the new food label to make the best choices for your own diet.

Let the Fat Fit the Diet

First, determine your daily calorie needs. A moderately active (30-60 minutes of exercise three times a week) adult needs about 15 calories per pound to maintain his or her weight. A less active person would need fewer calories and a more active person would need more.

Second, adapt fat goals to correspond with calorie needs. Total fat should be 30 percent or less of calories (one gram of fat contains 9 calories).

Now, to determine your recommended daily fat intake, follow this formula:

15 x body weight (in pounds) x .3 (30%) / 9 = recommended grams of fat per day

5 Health Dangers of High Fructose Corn Syrup

by Dr. Edward Group DC, NP, DACBN, DCBCN, DABFM Published on July 8, 2010, Last Updated on April 29, 2015

Since the late 1980s, HFCS has replaced regular table sugar, honey, and similar sweeteners. Prolonged consumption of HFCS is the topic of debate and, like other genetically modified products, may be bad for your health. A number of studies conducted over the past few decades indicate consumption of HFCS is connected with some health concerns.

1. Significant Risk of Weight Gain and Obesity
A study conducted by Princeton University [1], found that rats that were fed HFCS gained fat 300% more quickly than those fed an equal (or slightly larger) serving of fruit-derived sugar.

2. Increased Risk of Developing Type-2 Diabetes
Consumption of high-fructose corn syrup can lead to a huge increase in the likelihood of developing diabetes [2]. This life-long condition can be avoided in most cases. Excessive amounts of soda, energy drinks and junk-food aren't worth losing a foot or going blind for.

3. Hypertension and Elevated "Bad" Cholesterol Levels

High-fructose doesn't just make your body fat, it also makes your heart fat. There is a strong link between the irresponsible consumption of high fructose corn syrup and elevated triglyceride and LDL (bad cholesterol) levels [3]. Together, these can cause arterial plaque build-up and lead to heart problems including hypertension, heart disease, and even stroke.

4. High Fructose Corn Syrup and Liver Damage

This is a big one. Like anything else you eat or drink, your liver, gallbladder, and kidneys, processes HFCS. And it's especially destructive to your liver. When combined with a sedentary lifestyle, permanent liver scarring can occur [4]. This greatly diminishes the organ's ability to process out toxins and, over time, can lead to an expansive range of other negative health concerns. Another study suggests that HFCS may also cause fatty liver [5].

5. Mercury Exposure from HFCS

Did you know high fructose corn syrup is often loaded with alarmingly high levels of mercury? One study found mercury in over 50% of samples tested [6]. Mercury exposure can result in irreversible brain and nervous system damage – especially in young, growing bodies. Way too many foods aimed at children are LOADED with high fructose corn syrup!

Alternatives to High Fructose Corn Syrup

The dangers of high fructose corn syrup are both numerous and severe, if it's in your diet, remove it. Some estimate more than one-third of the American food supply has been polluted by this trash. I urge you to read product labels and avoid those with HFCS. Replace HFCS with raw honey for sweetening needs.

References:

1. Hilary Parker. A sweet problem: Princeton researchers find that high-fructose corn syrup prompts considerably more weight gain. Princeton University. 2010 March 22.
2. American Chemical Society. Soda Warning-high-fructose corn syrup linked to diabetes, new study suggests. ScienceDaily 23 Aug. 2007.
3. Jennifer K. Nelson R.D.,L.D. What is high-fructose corn syrup? What are the health concerns? Mayo Clinic. 2012 September 27.
4. Duke University Medical Center. High fructose corn syrup linked to liver scarring, research suggests. ScienceDaily. 23 Mar. 2010.
5. Laura G. Sánchez-Lozada, Wei Mu, Carlos Roncal, Yuri Y. Sautin, Manal Abdelmalek, Sirirat Reungjui, MyPhuong Le, Takahiko Nakagawa, Hui Y. Lan, Xuequing Yu, Richard J. Johnson. Comparison of free fructose and glucose to sucrose in the ability to cause fatty liver. European Journal of Nutrition. 2010 February. vol. 49 issue 1, pp. 1-9.
6. Dufault R, LeBlanc B, Schnoll R, Cornett C, Schweitzer L, Wallinga D, Hightower J, Patrick L, Lukiw WJ. Mercury from chlor-alkali plants: measured concentrations in food product sugar. Environ Health. 2009 Jan 26;8:2. doi: 10.1186/1476-069X-8-2.

MSG!!!

Again, you be the judge. In an effort to stay out of the courtroom, I am not going to tell you this product is the DEVIL. You must make the choice on your own, but from a fat person to more fat people, we eat a lot more of this product then the skinny people of the world. Just saying

The Dangers of Monosodium Glutamate

The problems associated with processed foods continue to grow. Our overabundance of these items has left a society struggling with poor nutrition and overall health. Information on the food additive monosodium glutamate, or MSG, needs to be shared to protect the American family.

MSG is a flavor enhancer traditionally used in Chinese food, but found today in many foods like breakfast sausages and potato chips. Understanding the pitfalls of MSG can be very confusing. Glutamate is a naturally occurring amino acid that the body uses and needs. The synthetic manipulation and processing of glutamate produces a form that is not found in nature. Proven by studying many other areas, particularly hormone medications, attempting to recreate a product of nature often produces less than desirable results. MSG has been labeled an excitotoxin because it is thought to have the ability to overstimulate cells to death. Many people link headaches, flushing, poor attention and other symptoms, as well as diseases like fibromyalgia, to MSG intake.

Research on MSG has varied, and conventional medicine lacks in understanding what many patients have already found. Research has documented several effects related to MSG, including burning sensations of the mouth, head and neck, weakness of the arms or legs, headaches and upset stomach approximately 15 minutes after the MSG is consumed [Source: Metcalfe]. Further research again points to problems such as flushing, headaches and hives or allergic-type reactions with the skin [Source: Izikson, Gladstein, Simon]. Other reports suggest that there is really no link between MSG and these symptoms, though this data seems to be wavering [Source: Fernstrom, Lawrence]. In fact, a double blind study (where both researchers and test subjects were not aware who was getting a real test or a fake test) found that MSG exposure caused muscle tightness, fatigue, numbness or tingling, and flushing [Source: Yang]. One study in mice concluded that injections of MSG produced obesity, inactivity and many other hormone fluctuations [Source: Lorden]. Respected neurosurgeon Russell Blaylock, M.D., even wrote a book on the subject, *Excitotoxins: The Taste That Kills.*

One of the most important factors in MSG research is that some of the effects can occur very quickly while others, that are perhaps much more detrimental, might be more cumulative over time with subsequent exposure. For example, a study done with animals found that MSG exposure over a period of 3-6 months led to significant risk for damage to the retinas of the eyes [Source: Ohguro]. These changes were not seen right away in the study, demonstrating that studies on MSG using 1-2 doses might miss many of the potential long-term effects associated with MSG intake.

MSG comes in many processed foods and snacks. Similar to high fructose corn syrup and partially hydrogenated oils, consumers need to get in the habit of looking for monosodium glutamate. MSG does not occur naturally in whole foods, so you do not have to worry about it in apples or bananas. Manufacturers are required to state if MSG is included in products on their food content label. Unfortunately, it might fall under different titles, making it very difficult to keep up with what foods contain the additive. MSGmyth.com lists other names for MSG, including monopotassium glutamate and vegetable protein extract, and several additives that contain various amounts of MSG.

Everyone will not be affected the same by MSG, and perhaps some will experience no problems at all. The uncertain and somewhat frightening aspect of this compound is that it can cause a variety of symptoms over time that can lead to much greater, more permanent problems. It could also be argued that small amounts in any one food will not be a problem, but if small amounts are in several common foods that are consumed every day, the problem moves to a much graver scale.

What is MSG? Is it bad for you?

Answers from Katherine Zeratsky, R.D., L.D.

Monosodium glutamate (MSG) is a flavor enhancer commonly added to Chinese food, canned vegetables, soups and processed meats. The Food and Drug Administration (FDA) has classified MSG as a food ingredient that's "generally recognized as safe," but its use remains controversial. For this reason, when MSG is added to food, the FDA requires that it be listed on the label.

MSG has been used as a food additive for decades. Over the years, the FDA has received many anecdotal reports of adverse reactions to foods containing MSG. These reactions — known as MSG symptom complex — include:

- Headache
- Flushing
- Sweating
- Facial pressure or tightness
- Numbness, tingling or burning in the face, neck and other areas
- Rapid, fluttering heartbeats (heart palpitations)
- Chest pain
- Nausea
- Weakness

However, researchers have found no definitive evidence of a link between MSG and these symptoms. Researchers acknowledge, though, that a small percentage of people may have short-term reactions to MSG. Symptoms are usually mild and don't require treatment. The only way to prevent a reaction is to avoid foods containing MSG.

Autolyzed Yeast	Calcium Caseinate	Gelatin
Glutamate	Glutamic Acid	Hydrolyzed Protein
Monopotassium Glutamate	Monosodium Glutamate	Sodium Caseinate
Textured Protein	Yeast Extract	Yeast Food
Yeast Nutrient		

These ingredients OFTEN contain MSG or create MSG during processing:10

Flavors and Flavorings	Seasonings	Natural Flavors and Flavorings	Natural Pork Flavoring	Natural Beef Flavoring
Natural Chicken Flavoring	Soy Sauce	Soy Protein Isolate	Soy Protein	Bouillon
Stock	Broth	Malt Extract	Malt Flavoring	Barley Malt
Anything Enzyme Modified	Carrageenan	Maltodextrin	Pectin	Enzymes
Protease	Corn Starch	Citric Acid	Powdered Milk	Anything Protein Fortified
	Anything Ultra-Pasteurized			

So, if you do eat processed foods, please remember to be on the lookout for these many hidden names for MSG.

GMO? Do you see a pattern yet? Coincident or not? Remember my rant earlier about natural or nothing? Where does genetically modified organism's fit into that sentence? So, before the bull shit starts flying and the Bibles come out for my next statement, here I go anyway. Why do we feel that we need to make everything better than we thought it was in the first place? MONEY!! So instead of eating a product given to us by God, in its natural form. We found ways to dissect it, break it down, make it get bigger yield more product so we could make more money off it. Again, here is some information to chew on and see if it affects you.

- GMO foods: What you need to know

- Why is there so much fuss over genetically modified ingredients? This will help you sift through the facts.
- Published: February 26, 2015 03:20 PMFoods made with canola oil, corn, or soy often contain GMOs.
- It's a growing controversy: Should GMO foods always be labeled so consumers are aware that the product contains genetically modified ingredients?
- GMOs—or genetically modified organisms—are created in a lab by altering the genetic makeup of a plant or an animal. Ninety-two percent of Americans believe that GMO foods—widely found in kitchens across the country—should be labeled before they're sold, according to a recent nationally representative survey of 1,004 people from the Consumer Reports National Research Center. (Last year our tests discovered that GMOs were present in many packaged foods, such as breakfast cereals, chips, baking mixes, and protein bars.)
- Demand for non-GMO foods has skyrocketed: In 2013, sales of non-GMO products that were either certified organic (by law, organic products can't be made with GMO ingredients) or that carried the "Non-GMO Project Verified" seal increased by 80 percent, according to the Nutrition Business Journal. It has prompted a growing number of companies to avoid using GMOs in new products or to voluntarily reformulate existing ones so that they can sport reliable non-GMO labels. PepsiCo, for example, sells Stacy's Simply Naked bagel and pita chips with the Non-GMO Project Verified seal; General Mills, which introduced a non-GMO original Cheerios cereal early last year, also has the non-GMO product lines Cascadian Farm and Food Should Taste Good.
- Yet GMO labeling has become a hot-button issue: Vermont passed a GMO labeling law last April. Last fall, the question of whether food manufacturers should be required to list GMO ingredients on their product labels was put to voters in Colorado and Oregon. On both sides were strong arguments and a lot of money spent—mostly on the part of food and chemical industry opponents to labeling. (In the Colorado election, for example, they outspent labeling supporters by about 16 to 1.) The measure was rejected in Colorado, and it failed in Oregon by a razor-thin margin in a recount—837 votes.

In an interesting twist, some food companies that expressed strong opposition to such mandatory labeling are the same ones turning out new non-GMO products. "They are experimenting, in case labeling does become mandatory and boosts demand for non-GMOs," says Nathan Hendricks, Ph.D., an agricultural economist at Kansas State University. "Of course, they may do this without too much fanfare to avoid raising questions about why they're removing GMOs from some of their products but not others."

With so many voices in the conversation and products on the market, how can you make buying decisions that are best for you and your family? Our Q&A helps you separate fact from fiction.

Are GMOs bad for my health?
Those who support using GMOs point out that Americans have been eating foods containing them for more than 15 years and that there's no credible evidence that people have been harmed. But saying there's no evidence of harm isn't the same as saying they've been proved safe. "The contention that GMOs pose no risks to human health can't be supported by studies that have measured a time frame that is too short to determine the effects of exposure over a lifetime," says Robert Gould, M.D., president of the board of Physicians for Social Responsibility.

A joint commission of the World Health Organization and the Food and Agriculture Organization of the United Nations has established a protocol for evaluating the safety of GMOs, which it says have the potential to introduce toxins and new allergens (or increase levels of existing ones), or cause nutritional changes in foods and other unexpected effects. Other developed nations have used those guidelines in their mandatory premarket safety assessments for genetically modified organisms. But the Food and Drug Administration doesn't require any safety assessment of genetically engineered crops, though it invites companies to provide data for a voluntary safety review.

Animal studies—commonly used to help assess human health risks—have suggested that GMOs might cause damage to the immune system, liver, and kidneys. More studies are needed to determine long-term effects. And the ability of researchers to track potential health effects of GMOs in the human population is hampered by the absence of labeling. "Physicians need to know what their patients are eating," Gould says. "If your patient has a problem with food allergies or other side effects that may be related to GMOs, it's difficult to identify any links unless these foods are labeled."

Why the labeling debate?
GMO labeling is mandatory in more than 60 countries but not in the U.S. Opponents to mandatory labeling here often say that it unfairly implies that foods with genetically engineered ingredients are unsafe. Those in favor of mandatory labels—including Consumers Union, the advocacy arm of Consumer Reports—argue that even if the jury is still out on the health impact of GMOs, shoppers have a right to know what's in their food. "Producers already must label foods that are frozen, from concentrate, homogenized, or irradiated," says Jean Halloran, director of food-policy initiatives at Consumers Union. "GMO labeling is one more piece of helpful information."

It's not surprising that much of the opposition to GMO labeling comes from GMO seed manufacturers and the food industry, who have spent a lot of money to get their position out to the public. Among those contributing the most to oppose the Colorado measure were Coca-Cola, DuPont, Kraft Foods, Monsanto (which produces seeds for GMO crops), and PepsiCo. The Grocery Manufacturers Association, the Snack Food Association, the International Dairy Foods Association, and the National Association of Manufacturers have filed a lawsuit to overturn Vermont's labeling law.

Which foods contain GMOs?
The vast majority of corn, soy, canola, and sugar beets grown in the U.S. are now genetically engineered, and they are often used as ingredients in processed foods.

The food industry is also pushing to further expand the use of genetic engineering. A new form of salmon that is genetically altered to grow to maturity twice as fast as wild salmon is currently undergoing a safety review by the Food and Drug Administration. If approved, it would be the first genetically engineered animal to be marketed.

The Department of Agriculture recently approved a potato that is genetically engineered to resist bruising and to have potentially lower levels of acrylamide, a suspected human carcinogen that the vegetable can produce when it is cooked at the high temperatures used to make potato chips and French fries. The FDA hasn't completed a voluntary safety review for the new GMO potato yet, but McDonald's has stated that it is sticking to its current policy of using only non-GMO potatoes for its fries.

Do GMOs harm the environment?
One main selling point for crops containing GMOs has been that they reduce the use of pesticides. The use of insecticides (which kill bugs) has declined since these crops were introduced in the mid-1990s, but the use of herbicides (which kill weeds) has soared.

The majority of corn, soybeans, and other GMO crops grown in the U.S. are genetically engineered to be resistant to glyphosate, a weed killer better known as Roundup. Roundup is made by Monsanto, which also produces the seeds that enable crops to survive being doused with the herbicide. Since that technology was introduced in 1996, there has been almost a tenfold increase in the use of the herbicide, as illustrated in this graph from the U.S. Geological Survey.

That in turn created an epidemic of super-weeds, which have quickly evolved to become immune to glyphosate. A survey conducted by Stratus Agri-Marketing in 2012 found that almost half of farmers throughout the U.S. are now battling the crop-choking plants.

The solution proposed by the biotech industry? Creating a new generation of crops that are genetically altered to be immune to glyphosate and to other herbicides that are capable of killing the glyphosate-resistant super-weeds. Dow AgroSciences recently got the green light from federal officials to sell its new Enlist brand of GMO corn and soybeans, which are both engineered to be resistant to glyphosate as well as to an herbicide known as 2,4-D.

The USDA has estimated that Dow's new GMO corn and soybean crops would at least triple the use of 2,4-D and could lead to an almost sevenfold increase over the next five years. "Since this is likely to make even more weeds immune to both Roundup and 2,4-D, this 'solution' to the super-weed problem makes about as much sense as pouring gasoline on a fire to put it out," says Charles Benbrook, Ph.D., a research professor at Washington State University who also serves on a USDA advisory committee on agricultural biotechnology.

Significant increases in the use of these herbicides could potentially affect consumers' health as well, because residue from the chemicals can end up in food crops. In a letter to the Environmental Protection Agency raising concerns about increased exposure to 2,4-D that would result from approval of Dow's new GMO corn and soy, a group of 70 scientists, doctors, and other health professionals pointed out that studies in humans have reported associations between exposure to the herbicide and increased risks of non-Hodgkins lymphoma, birth defects, and other reproductive problems.

Will GMO labeling drive up grocery prices?
Mandatory labeling that informs consumers about whether their food contains GMOs would add less than a penny a day to their grocery bills, according to a recent analysis of existing studies commissioned by Consumers Union and conducted by the independent economic research firm ECONorthwest.

Opponents of labeling cite industry-financed studies suggesting that food prices would soar, boosting a typical family of four's spending at the supermarket by $400 to $800 per year. But the Consumers Union analysis found that the median cost that might be passed on to consumers was just $2.30 per person annually—or $9.20 for a family of four.

Why such a big difference? The industry's estimate assumes that if consumers know that a product contains GMOs, they'll perceive it negatively and won't buy it. Food producers would then, in many cases, replace GMOs with much more expensive organic ingredients, and food prices would escalate.

But in countries where GMO labeling is required—including many where American food companies sell their products—food prices haven't increased as a result of mandatory labeling. And as our recent GMO testing showed, food products don't have to contain all-organic ingredients to qualify as non-GMO.

Did you know?
Because corn and soybeans are the most widely planted genetically modified crops in the U.S., it's not surprising that you'd find GMO corn in tortilla chips or GMO soy in some meat substitutes. But those genetically engineered ingredients also pop up in places you might not expect. Some spices and seasoning mixes contain GMO corn and soy. And soft-drink ingredients that might be derived from genetically modified corn include not only corn syrup but also the artificial sweetener aspartame, glucose, citric acid, and colorings such as beta-carotene and riboflavin.
Products and politics: GMO info at your fingertips
The upside of all the publicity generated by the GMO debate is increased awareness among consumers, who are often moved to reach out to companies to find out what's in their food, says Megan Westgate, executive director of the Non-GMO Project. It certifies through third-party testing that products carrying its seal qualify as non-GMO.
"I don't think people realize how much power they really have in the marketplace," Westgate says. The Non-GMO Project Verified seal, launched in 2010, now appears on more than 22,000 products that represent $8.5 billion in annual sales at retailers across the country. "At least 200 companies that have come to us to become non-GMO verified have said they were prompted to make that change because of calls or letters they'd gotten from consumers."
To help you exercise that power, the Non-GMO Project recently launched a free iPhone app, available on iTunes, that allows you to search for products verified as non-GMO. If your favorite food isn't listed, the app directs you to a form to let the manufacturer know that you would like it to be. Consumers who want

to avoid GMOs can also express their preferences in the marketplace by buying certified organic foods. Consumers Union, the policy arm of Consumer Reports, favors labeling and premarket safety testing of GMO foods and supports state bills and measures to that end. We also strongly oppose the introduction of a food- and chemical-industry supported federal bill that would preempt all state GMO food-labeling laws and would allow the "natural" label to be used on GMO foods.

1. "Center for Food Safety | Issues | GE Food Labeling | International Labeling Laws." *Center for Food Safety.* N.p., n.d. Web.
2. Langer, Gary. "Poll: Skepticism of Genetically Modified Foods." *ABC News.* ABC News Network, 19 June 2015. Web.
3. Fernandez-Cornejo, Jorge, and Seth James Wechsler. "USDA ERS – Adoption of Genetically Engineered Crops in the U.S.: Recent Trends in GE Adoption." *USDA ERS – Adoption of Genetically Engineered Crops in the U.S.: Recent Trends in GE Adoption.* United States Department of Agriculture, Economic Research Service, 09 July 2015. Web.
4. Leader, Jessica. "Monsanto Wins Lawsuit Filed By U.S. Organic Farmers Worried About Seed Contamination." *The Huffington Post.* TheHuffingtonPost.com, 10 June 2013. Web.
5. Duke, S.O., & Powles, S.B. (2009). "Glyphosate-resistant crops and weeds: Now and in the future." *AgBioForum,* 12(3&4), 346-357.
6. Kustin, Mary Ellen. "Glyphosate Is Spreading Like a Cancer Across the U.S." *EWG.* Environmental Working Group, 07 Apr. 2015. Web.
7. Mortensen DA, Egan JF, Maxwell BD, Ryan MR, Smith RG. "Navigating a critical juncture for sustainable weed management." *BioScience.* 2012;62(1):75-84.
8. "Newsroom." *Agent Orange: Background on Monsanto's Involvement.* N.p., n.d. Web.

RBGH, what is it good for? Profit

Here is the next contestant on this could have made me fat!!! This is another product the FDA has deemed as safe, but you be the judge of that after you peruse the following studies. I mentioned this several times throughout the book, I am a product of the sixties, but my kids are products of the 80's and 90's so we ate a lot of the same food and drank the same milk. I graduated high school with a size 10 shoe. I was 6'2 190 at graduation. My son graduated high school 6'4 185 with a 14.5 shoe. Just saying Coincidence?

FACT SHEET Recombinant Bovine Growth Hormone (rBGH or rBST) Its Documented Harm to Cows Background
The FDA approved the use of recombinant bovine growth hormone (rBGH or rBST) in dairy cows in 1993. This was done over the widespread objections of farmers, public health advocates and animal welfare agencies. This genetically engineered hormone was developed by Monsanto and sold to Elanco, a division of the Eli Lilly drug company, in 2008. Its trade name is Posilac.®
There is overwhelming documented evidence that rBGH increases the rates of physical harm to cows. This paper summarizes the case against the use of rBGH on animal welfare grounds and reinforces the call to disallow it.
FDA Posilac® Package Insert
Although the FDA allowed rBGH to be commercialized, it acknowledged that it increased the rates of 16 harmful physical effects on cows and required an insert, listing the following conditions, be placed in every package sold. These include:
Reproductive Effects: Reduced pregnancy rates, increase in days open, increased incidence of retained placenta, decreased gestation length and birth weight of calves Increased rate of clinical mastitis and Increased rate of subclinical mastitis (somatic cell count) Increased body temperature unrelated to illness (heat stress) Increase in digestive disorders, such as indigestion, bloat and diarrhea Increase in reduced feed intake (of-feed) Increased numbers of enlarged hocks and lesions and increased numbers of foot disorders Increased number of injection site reactions – swelling Reductions in hemoglobin and hematocrit values
FDA Adverse Drug Reaction Reports   After rBGH was approved, farmers submitted reports to the FDA describing harm the drug had caused to their cows. These included all of the above, plus others, such as abortions, birth defects, increased twinning rates and lameness.
These harmful effects are widespread. From 1994 to 2005, the FDA received 2,408 adverse drug reaction reports from farmers that described harmful effects to cows injected with rBGH. (Freedom of Information Act documents received from FDA, Sept. 2010) There are currently about 65,000 dairy farmers in the U.S.
USDA Reports
The USDA periodically issues reports on the state of American agriculture, including dairy. Their Dairy 2002 Report was clear on rBGH:
"Dairy producers have expressed concerns about (r)bST use. These concerns include: animal health . . . and public health concerns . . . Dairy producers that were not currently using bST were asked to describe

their reason for not implementing a bST program . . . cost and animal health were major concerns specifically identified in all regions . . ."

Academic Studies

Henry Ann and Leslie Butler have done several studies on why farmers started and later dis adopted use of rBGH. Their 1997-98 study found "Many (farmers) . . . had problems like mastitis, lameness, loss of condition, and lowered immune system functions which they attributed to rbST use." Their 2008 report on disadoption rates in California found that 15% of farmers cited high veterinary costs as "very important" in their decision to stop using rBGH. (Henry An and Leslie Butler, "Update on rBST Use in the California Dairy Industry," Giannini Foundation of Agricultural Economics – University of California, 2008)

Canada and European Union Bans on rBGH Use

Although scientists in Canada and the European Union expressed human health concerns about rBGH, specifically cancer and antibiotic resistance, the official reason that both banned rBGH was harm to cows. The Canadian Veterinary Medical Association Expert Panel of rbST determined that mastitis increased by 25%, infertility by 18%, lameness by 50% and culling (slaughter) by 20-25%. (Report of Canadian Veterinary Medical Association Expert Panel on rbST. Prepared for Health Canada, November, 1998. At: http://www.hc-sc.gc.ca/dhp-mps/vet/issues-enjeux/rbst-stbr/rep_cvma-rap_acdv_tc-tm-eng.php). Health Canada announced in January 1999 that "it had to reject the request for approval to use rbST in Canada, as it presents a sufficient and unacceptable threat to the safety of dairy cows." (Institute of Food Science and Technology Information Statement on Bovine Somatotropin. 2004, p. 5 at: www.ifst.org/document.aspx?id=113)

A scientific committee in the EU found rBGH use led to "painful and debilitating" conditions in cows and "Therefore from the point of view of animal welfare, including health, the Scientific /Committee on Animal Health and Animal Welfare is of the opinion that (r)BST should not be used in dairy cows." (Report on Animal Welfare Aspects of Use of Recombinant Bovine Somatotropin. Report of the Scientific Committee on Animal Health and Animal Welfare. March 10, 1999. At: http://ec.europa.eu/food/fs/sc/scah/out21_en.pdf)

Organizational Stances

Virtually every major animal welfare organization in the U.S. opposes rBGH. This includes the Humane Society of the U.S. (HSUS), Humane Farming Association and Farm Sanctuary. According to Miyun Park, former Vice President of Farm Animal Welfare of HSUS, "It's simply wrong to inject cows with a substance like rBGH that increases painful and debilitating diseases like mastitis and lameness." ("Know Your Milk", Oregon Physicians for Social Responsibility, 2010)

Both the National Family Farm Coalition and Family Farm Defenders oppose rBGH. John Kinsman, president of the Family Farm Defenders, stated "The FDA"s approval . . . did not even consider the demonstrated health impacts on dairy cows or the potential risks to human consumers."

Voices of the Farmers Themselves – A small sample:

Tillamook dairy farmer Dick Heathershaw . . . "quit using the product (rBGH) after noticing cows were splitting out in the pelvic area, were growing hooves at an accelerated rate and were experiencing unusually high levels of abscesses . . . „we thought we were seeing things in our cow's health-wise that we didn't like and that we hadn't seen before. "" (Capital Press, Feb. 25, 2005)

" „It's like steroids for athletes, " said Stephen H. Taylor, New Hampshire's Commissioner of Agriculture, Markets and Food and a dairy farmer himself. He said he had tried the hormone but it put stress on his cows and made them thinner." (New York Times, Oct. 7, 2006)

". . . most Country Classic farmers weren't keen on growth hormone because of the potential harm to their stock. The word among farmers was that growth hormone boosted milk production in the short term but shortened the cow's productive life." (Billings, MT Gazette, Sept. 13, 2008)

-Fact Sheet developed by Rick North, Oregon Physicians for Social Responsibility, November 2010

8 Shocking Facts about Bovine Growth Hormone

by Dr. Edward Group DC, NP, DACBN,

Since bovine growth hormone received FDA approval in 1993, three disturbing health trends have emerged. Cancer cases continue to increase; obesity has become an epidemic and early onset puberty has become the norm. [1] [2] [3] Related? Maybe, maybe not. You can be the judge as you read through the following 8 facts about the substance known as BGH, or rBGH. Whatever conclusion you arrive at, you'll probably agree that keeping this substance far away from you and your family is good practice.

1. Bovine Growth Hormone is a GMO

Monsanto created rBGH to stimulate milk production in cows. At least that's the nice way of saying it. Bovine growth hormone occurs naturally in cows; the same way human growth hormone occurs naturally in humans. To make it more "effective", Monsanto genetically modified BGH to create recombinant Bovine Growth Hormone, or rBGH or rBST (recombinant bovine somatotrophin). This more potent GMO version of BGH is not a naturally occurring substance and does more than increase ol' Bessie's milk production.

2. It's Banned in the European Union and Around the World

Originally approved by many countries shortly after its release, rBGH has since been banned by the European Union, Canada, Australia, Japan, New Zealand, and Israel. [4] Most of these bans went into effect in 2000, some earlier. It didn't take their scientists long to figure out this stuff isn't quite right.

3. Medical Experts Have Declared It Unsafe

In 2007, Dr. Samuel Epstein exposed the dangers of rBGH in his book *What's in your Milk?* This book reveals the science, politics, and corporate greed behind the creation and approval of rBGH. [5] Since then, many milk producers have decided to sell only rBGH-free milk; and Monsanto sold its rBGH business unit to Eli Lilly. [6] But don't be fooled, it's still out there and likely to remain out there and in the food supply until a full ban is established.

4. A Human danger: Contains Insulin Like Growth Factor (IGF-1)

Milk from cows treated with rBGH contains higher levels of IGF-1. The American Cancer Society reports early studies linked IGF-1 as a contributor to tumor development, specifically breast, prostate and colorectal cancers. [7] While research has not clarified the connection, continuing efforts support these studies...

5. Links to Various Types of Cancer

Insulin like growth factor has a multitude of problems. A recently published scientific review focused on the relation of IGF-1 (and IGF-2) to breast cancer tumor formation. These insulin growth factors are known to stimulate cell differentiation. It appears IGFs have a unique interaction with estrogen which may contribute to tumor development in women. [8]

A 2013 study evaluated the relation of IFG and prostate cancer. Little if any IGF was observed in healthy prostate tissue. Advanced tumors demonstrated a high presence of IGF-1, while smaller localized prostate cancer tumors showed a lesser density of IGF-1. Ultimately the study concluded higher concentrations of IGF-1 do have a correlation to the presence of prostate cancer. [9]

Like prostate cancer, advanced colorectal cancers have shown a direct relationship with higher levels of IGF-1. One particular study demonstrated higher levels in men, patients over 60 and those with cancers stemming from damage to the mucus layer of the colon. The researchers determined IGF-1 levels can indicate and help identify the presence of colorectal cancers. [10]

6. Linked to Lung Cancer Too?

Although not one of the original cancers linked to insulin like growth factor, recent research from China has found that IGF-1 plays a significant role in non-small cell lung cancer. Lung cancer patients in this study had much higher blood serum levels of IGF-1 than the control group. [11] While this study is relatively new, it does suggest IGF-1 may play a larger role in cancers than previously thought. It also raises additional concerns and questions about the role of increased consumption of IGF as a result of genetically modified cows.

7. Diabetes as a Result of BGH?

FDA and Monstanto scientists determined the rBGH used on cows wouldn't transfer or affect humans, especially through milk. They also stated that bovine growth hormone wouldn't affect humans even if ingested. A case documented in 2011 suggests otherwise.

A 33-year-old man found himself in the ER reporting a range of symptoms including nausea, headaches, blurry vision, and more. In the course of the examination, the patient admitted taking anabolic steroids — which included bovine growth hormone. (Apparently, bodybuilders know something more about the effect of bovine growth hormone on humans than government and corporate researchers!) As a result of the use, he began a new life with diabetes. [12]

While this is a very unique case, it does show that bovine growth hormone, whether introduced via milk (which we've been told it won't be) or through other means can have serious effects on human health.

8. Other Side Effects: Milk Contamination, Mastitis, and Antibiotics

Cows given rBGH are more likely to develop mastitis, an inflammation and infection of mammary tissue. Early studies found this led to bacteria and potential pus in milk. While laws prohibit distribution of contaminated milk, the simple fact is that milk from cows treated with rBGH are more likely to suffer contamination than others. This problem was one of the reasons the European Union and other countries banned it. [4]

rBGH also causes a wide range of health problems for cows, requiring the use of antibiotics. Fortunately, most producers label their milk, so it is easy to find non-rBGH/rBST milk. Of course, the easiest way is to buy organic or raw. Better yet — choose organic goat's milk.

References:
1. American Institute for Cancer Research. Number of US Cancer Cases Expected to Rise 55 Percent Higher by 2030. (last accessed (2014-01-02)
2. Medical News Today. US obesity rates on the rise: 113 million by 2022. (last accessed (2014-01-02)
3. Elizabeth Weil. New York Times. Puberty Before Age 10: A New "Normal"? (last accessed (2014-01-02)
4. Food Safety – From the Farm to the Fork. Report on Public Health Aspects of the Use of Bovine Somatotrophin – 15-16 March 199. (last accessed (2014-01-02)
5. World-Wire. What's in Your Milk? (last accessed (2014-01-02)
6. New York Times. Eli Lilly to Buy Monsanto's Dairy Cow Hormone for $300 Million. (last accessed (2014-01-02)
7. American Cancer Society. Recombinant Bovine Growth Hormone. (last accessed (2014-01-02)
8. Hawsawi Y, El-Gendy R, Twelves C, Speirs V, Beattie J. Insulin-like growth factor – Oestradiol crosstalk and mammary gland tumourigenesis. Biochim Biophys Acta. 2013 Nov 2. pii: S0304-419X(13)00047-4. doi: 10.1016/j.bbcan.2013.10.005.
9. Savvani A, Petraki C, Msaouel P, Diamanti E, Xoxakos I, Koutsilieris M. IGF-IEc expression is associated with advanced clinical and pathological stage of prostate cancer. Anticancer Res. 2013 Jun;33(6):2441-5.
10. Kukliski A, Kamocki Z, Cepowicz D, Gryko M, Czyewska J, Pawlak K, Kdra B. Relationships between insulin-like growth factor I and selected clinico-morphological parameters in colorectal cancer patients. Pol Przegl Chir. 2011 May;83(5):250-7. doi: 10.2478/v10035-011-0039-z.
11. Wang Z, Wang Z, Liang Z, Liu J, Shi W, Bai P, Lin X, Magaye R, Zhao J. Expression and clinical significance of IGF-1, IGFBP-3, and IGFBP-7 in serum and lung cancer tissues from patients with non-small cell lung cancer. Onco Targets Ther. 2013 Oct 16;6:1437-44. doi: 10.2147/OTT.S51997.
12. Geraci MJ, Cole M, Davis P. New onset diabetes associated with bovine growth hormone and testosterone abuse in a young bodybuilder. Hum Exp Toxicol. 2011 Dec;30(12):2007-12. doi: 10.1177/0960327111408152. Epub 2011 May 9.

Fast Food, how fast you want to die? That's not fair, remember I did spend almost 20 years of my life in that business, it does have its benefits. Where else is our youth of America going to learn to say "do you want fries with that" and not learn how to count back change without a calculator? Think about it, you are trusting your life and the lives of your family on Bobby the burger flipper and Freddy the fry slinger. Your health is in great shape. Oh, wait don't forget about Debbie Diet Coke, you have to have something to wash all those calories down with. Right? Again, this is a lifestyle change we are talking about, there is nothing wrong with the food they are serving to you, other than it is unhealthy. Take a minute to peruse the literature I have provided for you. I found this in like two minutes on the internet. But Big Sexy, it tastes so good though. Real food can taste just as good if you give it a try!! Just saying.

Effects of fast food on the Body

Fast foods often contain too many calories and too little nutrition. If fast food is a regular component of your diet, you might find yourself struggling with weight problems and ill health.

Extra Calories

Insulin Resistance

High Blood Pressure

Bloating and Puffiness

Shortness of Breath

Depression

Dental Distress

Blood Sugar Spike

A Weighty Problem

High Cholesterol

Hard on the Heart

Headache

Acne

Effects of Fast Food on the Body

Food is fuel for your body. It has a direct impact on how you feel as well as on your overall health. Fast food isn't necessarily bad, but in many cases, it's highly processed and contains large amounts of carbohydrates, added sugar, unhealthy fats, and salt (sodium).

These foods are often high in calories yet offer little or no nutritional value. When fast food frequently replaces nutritious foods in your diet, it can lead to poor nutrition, poor health, and weight gain. Tests in lab animals have even shown a negative effect in short duration diets. Being overweight is a risk factor for a variety of chronic health problems including heart disease, diabetes, and stroke.

According to the Robert Wood Johnson Foundation, most people underestimate the number of calories they're eating in a fast-food restaurant. A 2013 study published in JAMA Pediatrics showed that children and adolescents take in more calories in fast food and other restaurants than at home. Eating at a restaurant added between 160 and 310 calories a day.

Digestive and Cardiovascular Systems

Many fast foods and drinks are loaded with carbohydrates and, consequently, a lot of calories. Your digestive system breaks carbs down into sugar (glucose), which it then releases into your bloodstream.

Your pancreas responds by releasing insulin, which is needed to transport sugar to cells throughout your body. As the sugar is absorbed, your blood sugar levels drop. When blood sugar gets low, your pancreas releases another hormone called glucagon. Glucagon tells the liver to start making use of stored sugars.

When everything is working in sync, blood sugar levels stay within a normal range. When you take in high amounts of carbs, it causes a spike in your blood sugar. That can alter the normal insulin response. Frequent spikes in blood sugar may be a contributing factor in insulin resistance and type 2 diabetes.

Sugar and Fat

Added sugars have no nutritional value but are high in calories. According to the American Heart Association, most Americans take in twice as much sugar as is recommended for optimal health. All those extra calories add up to extra weight, which is a contributing factor for getting heart disease.

Trans fats are a manufactured fat with no extra nutritional value. They're considered so unhealthy that some countries have banned their use. Often found in fast food, trans fats are known to raise LDL cholesterol levels. That's the undesirable kind of cholesterol. They can also lower HDL cholesterol, which is the so-called good cholesterol. Trans fats may also increase your risk of developing type 2 diabetes.

Sodium

Too much sodium causes your body to retain water, making you feel bloated and puffy. But that's the least of the damage overly salted foods can do. Sodium also can contribute to existing high blood pressure or enlarged heart muscle. If you have congestive heart failure, cirrhosis, or kidney disease, too much salt can contribute to a dangerous buildup of fluid. Excess sodium may also increase your risk for kidney stones, kidney disease, and stomach cancer.

High cholesterol and high blood pressure are among the top risk factors for heart disease and stroke.

Respiratory System

Obesity is associated with an increase in respiratory problems. Even without diagnosed medical conditions, obesity may cause episodes of shortness of breath or wheezing with little exertion. Obesity also can play a role in the development of sleep apnea, a condition in which sleep is continually disrupted by shallow breathing and asthma.

A recent study published in the journal Thorax suggests that children who eat fast food at least three times a week are at increased risk of asthma and rhinitis, which involves having a congested, drippy nose.

Central Nervous System

A study published in the journal Public Health Nutrition showed that eating commercial baked goods (doughnuts, croissants, and, yes, even bran muffins) and fast food (pizza, hamburgers, and hot dogs) may be linked to depression. The study determined that people who eat fast food are 51 percent more likely to develop depression than those who eat little to no fast food. It was also found that the more fast food study participants consumed, the more likely they were to develop depression.

A junk food diet could also affect your brain's synapses and the molecules related to memory and learning, according to a study published in the journal Nature. Animal tests have shown a similar effect. Rats fed a steady diet with over half the calories from fat (similar to a junk food diet) for just a few days had trouble completing a maze they had previously mastered in a 2009 study.

Skin and Bones

Chocolate and greasy foods are often blamed for acne, but they're not the real culprits. It's carbs that are to blame. According to the Mayo Clinic, because foods that are high in carbohydrates increase blood sugar levels, they may also trigger acne.

The study in Thorax showed a higher risk of eczema (inflamed, irritated patches of skin) among children with a diet high in fast food.

When you consume foods high in carbs and sugar, bacteria residing in your mouth produce acids. These acids can destroy tooth enamel, a contributing factor in dental cavities. When the enamel of your tooth is lost, it can't be replaced. Poor oral health has also been linked to other health problems.

Excess sodium may also increase your risk of developing osteoporosis (thin, fragile bones).

Effects on Society

According to the Centers for Disease Control and Prevention (CDC), the definition of obesity is when your body mass index (BMI) is 30.0 or higher. BMI is a calculation of your height and weight. You can calculate your BMI here. There's also a category referred to as "extreme obesity," which is defined as a BMI of 40. Across all race groups, one in three Americans is considered obese while one in 20 is considered extremely obese. Those statistics are higher in the black and Latino communities. Approximately 75 percent of people in these groups who are over age 20 are considered obese.

The Obesity Action Coalition (OAC) reports that the number of fast food outlets has doubled since 1970, a period during which the number of obese Americans also doubled. It's likely that many factors have contributed to the obesity epidemic, but the correlation between the availability of cheap and fattening fast food and national weight increase is stark. Obesity increases the likelihood of heart disease, high blood pressure, kidney disease, diabetes, joint problems, and more. In 2008, obesity-related medical costs were estimated at $147 billion. Diabetes alone was estimated to be responsible for $69 billion just in lost productivity. Numbers like these suggest that the costs of cheap fast food are surprisingly high.

Fast food is generally much higher in empty calories than other foods. It fills you up for awhile but doesn't give your body what it needs. Read more.

Fast food is generally much higher in empty calories than other foods. It fills you up for awhile but doesn't give your body what it needs. Read more.

A meal high in carbs means blood sugar levels can be expected to rise quickly. Read more.

A rise in blood sugar means more insulin is needed to process it. When that happens too often, it can interfere with your body's ability to use insulin effectively. Read more.

Food loaded with carbs, unhealthy fats, and sugars make it easy to tip the scales in the wrong direction. Overweight and obesity are associated with a multitude of health problems. Read more.

Excess salt and weight gain can make your blood pressure rise. Read more.

Fast foods can raise your bad cholesterol (LDL) while lowering the good (HDL), a double whammy. Read more.

Salt makes you retain water and can be blamed for some of that bloating and puffiness. Read more.

High cholesterol, high blood pressure, and obesity make your heart work harder and are among the leading causes of heart disease and stroke. Read more.

Studies show that obesity may contribute to breathing problems, including sleep apnea and asthma. Read more.

Fast food often contains ingredients that contribute to headaches. Read more.

The more fast food you eat, the more likely you are to develop depression, according to a recent study. Read more.

Greasy foods and chocolate don't really give you acne — it's all about the carbs. Read more.

All those sugars wreak havoc in your mouth, and cavities are sure to follow. Read more.

Article resources

- Adult BMI calculator. (2015, May 15). Retrieved from http://www.cdc.gov/healthyweight/assessing/bmi/adult_bmi/english_bmi_calculator/bmi_calculator.html
- All about cavities. (2012, August 6). Retrieved from http://www.simplestepsdental.com/SS/ihtSSPrint/r.WSIHW000/st.31845/t.32653/pr.3/c.354774.html

- Carbohydrates and blood sugar. (n.d.). Retrieved from http://www.hsph.harvard.edu/nutritionsource/carbohydrates/carbohydrates-and-blood-sugar/

- Chronic disease overview. (2015, August 26). Retrieved from http://www.cdc.gov/chronicdisease/overview/

- Consumers underestimate calories in fast-food meals. (n.d.). Retrieved from http://www.rwjf.org/en/library/articles-and-news/2013/05/consumers-underestimate-calories-in-fast-food-meals--teens-do-so.html

- Defining adult overweight and obesity. (2012, April 27). Retrieved from http://www.cdc.gov/obesity/adult/defining.html

- Diabetes myths. (2014, August 5). Retrieved from http://www.diabetes.org/diabetes-basics/myths/

- Diet for headache patients. (n.d.). Retrieved from http://www.stjohnprovidence.org/Migraine/HealthInfo/Diet/

- Effects of excess sodium on your health and appearance. (2014, April 10). Retrieved from http://www.heart.org/HEARTORG/GettingHealthy/NutritionCenter/HealthyDietGoals/The-Effects-of-Excess-Sodium-on-Your-Health-and-Appearance_UCM_454387_Article.jsp

- Ellwood P., Asher, M. I., Garcia-Marcos, L., Williams, H., Keil, U., Robertson, C., ... the ISAAC Phase III Study Group. (2012, November 1). Do fast foods cause asthma, rhinoconjunctivitis and eczema? Global findings from the International Study of Asthma and Allergies in Childhood (ISAAC) Phase Three [Abstract]. *Thorax.* Retrieved from http://thorax.bmj.com/content/early/2013/01/03/thoraxjnl-2012-202285.abstract

- Garcia, G., Sunil, T., & Hinojosa, P. (2012). The fast food and obesity link: Consumption patterns and severity of obesity. *Obesity Surgery, (22)*5, 810-818. Retrieved from http://www.ncbi.nlm.nih.gov/pubmed/22271359

- Gómez-Pinilla, F. (2008, July 1). Brain foods: The effects of nutrients on brain function. Retrieved from http://www.nature.com/nrn/journal/v9/n7/abs/nrn2421.html

- High-fat diet affects physical and memory abilities. (2009, August 1). Retrieved from http://www.cam.ac.uk/research/news/high-fat-diet-affects-physical-and-memory-abilities

- Mayo Clinic Staff. (2011, October 21). Acne: Causes. Retrieved from http://www.mayoclinic.org/diseases-conditions/acne/basics/causes/con-20020580

- Mayo Clinic Staff. (2013, May 11). Oral health: A window to your overall health. Retrieved from http://www.mayoclinic.org/healthy-living/adult-health/in-depth/dental/art-20047475

- National Institutes of Health. (2004, December 30). Eating at fast-food restaurants more than twice per week is associated with more weight gain and insulin resistance in otherwise healthy young adults [Press Release]. Retrieved from http://www.nih.gov/news/pr/dec2004/nhlbi-30.htm

- Obesity Action Coalition. Fast food – Is it the enemy? (n.d.). Retrieved from http://www.obesityaction.org/educational-resources/resource-articles-2/nutrition/fast-food-is-it-the-enemy

- Overweight and obesity in the U.S. (n.d.). Retrieved from http://frac.org/initiatives/hunger-and-obesity/obesity-in-the-us/

- Overweight and obesity statistics. (n.d.). Retrieved from http://www.niddk.nih.gov/health-information/health-statistics/Pages/overweight-obesity-statistics.aspx

- Powell, L. M., & Nguyen, B. T. (2013). Fast-food and full-service restaurant consumption among children and adolescents. *JAMA Pediatrics, 167*(1), 14-20. Retrieved from http://archpedi.jamanetwork.com/article.aspx?articleid=1389390

- Robbins J. M., Mallya G., Wagner A., & Buehler J. W. (2015, August 20). Prevalence, disparities, and trends in obesity and severe obesity among students in the School District of Philadelphia, Pennsylvania, 2006–2013. *Preventing Chronic Disease* 12. Retrieved from http://www.cdc.gov/Pcd/issues/2015/15_0185.htm

- Sánchez-Villegas, A., Toledo, E., de Irala, J., Ruiz-Canela, M., Pla-Vidal, J., & Martínez-González, M. A. (2011). Fast-food and commercial baked goods consumption and the risk of depression. *Public Health Nutrition,* *15*(03), 424. Retrieved from http://journals.cambridge.org/action/displayFulltext?type=6&fid=8480072&jid=PHN&volumeId=15&issueId=03&aid=8480071&bodyId=&membershipNumber=&societyETOCSession=&fulltextType=RA&fileId=S1368980011001856

- Sugar 101. (n.d.). Retrieved from http://www.heart.org/HEARTORG/GettingHealthy/NutritionCenter/HealthyEating/Sugar-101_UCM_306024_Article.jsp

- The cost of diabetes. (n.d.). Retrieved from http://www.diabetes.org/advocacy/news-events/cost-of-diabetes.html?referer=https://www.google.com/

- The effects of excess sodium on your health and appearance. (n.d.). Retrieved from http://www.heart.org/HEARTORG/GettingHealthy/NutritionCenter/HealthyDietGoals/The-Effects-of-Excess-Sodium-on-Your-Health-and-Appearance_UCM_454387_Article.jsp

- Trans fats. (2014, August 5). Retrieved from http://www.heart.org/HEARTORG/GettingHealthy/NutritionCenter/HealthyEating/Trans-Fats_UCM_301120_Article.jsp

- Zammit, C., Liddicoat, H., Moonsie, I., & Makker, H. (2010, October 20). Obesity and respiratory diseases. *International Journal of General Medicine*, 3, 335–343. Retrieved from http://www.ncbi.nlm.nih.gov/pmc/articles/PMC2990395/

Tick tock, tick tock, tick tock. One of the biggest adjustments I have had to make coming back to the mitten, is readjusting to family life. Not so much the first two meals of the day, because the first meal is between five and six am and no one is awake but me, as far as the second meal, if I need one. I am on my own for that one also. The third meal is the tricky one, notice I didn't say dinner? I still am working with my body to break the cycle of the establishment, so I feel better just numbering them. The issue comes in that my wife very regularly doesn't arrive home on a regular time schedule. It makes it difficult to establish a pattern for my body and stay cordial with my wife and her meal time. My wife works hard and I do my best to make sure that I prepare a good meal for her when she comes home, the issue comes in when it's ready and she is not. If it was up to me I would eat at 4:30 every day and she could fend for herself with the microwave, but I haven't had to resort to that yet!!! I know she doesn't do it on purpose, but it still messes with my bodies needs just the same. It's hard to build a trust with your body and not feed it when it is hungry, because you are waiting for someone else to arrive. You can rationalize with it all you want, but the fact remains you are putting your needs second and that hurts your trust with your body. Just saying

On the subject of time, why are we so impatient? Even instant, isn't fast enough for us in today's society. My buddy and I were in the car today and an old deer hunting song came on the radio. He made a smart assed comment about the song and the band that sang it. Then he had to bust out the fact that I had their album on a cassette tape back in the 80's when the song was first out. It made me think about the evolution of even the music industry over the past 25 years or so. Things started out on albums. Those are those black pancake thingies, no body uses anymore, for you skinny people playing along. Then we progressed to real to real, then eight track tapes, cassette tapes, cd's, mp3's then satellite radio, so we don't even need any additional devices to hear our favorite music. Sites like Pandora or Ihart Radio, where you can program your favorite songs to play. Going back to my Jetson's days, I thought by 2016 we would have the capability to go to our computers and punch up what we wanted to eat for dinner and it would magically appear for us on the table. Not quite there yet, but we can use our computers to look up the nutritional value of the food we are about to put into our bodies and create a good meal plan in the process. Just saying!

America, the land of opportunity: First of all, let me state for the record. America is the greatest country on the planet. Everyone hates us, because they want to be us. Too bad for them there is only one of us. Thank God for that as well, we are not talking about the skinnier healthy one of us either. There is a lot of us to go around. My wife and I had a candid conversation last night about some comments I made about the size of the people we saw at Logan's Steakhouse the other day. No I wasn't bashing fat people if that is what you are thinking. I was just commenting on how large some of the people were and that they didn't care about it. They still ordered pretty large meals and saved room for dessert. She was quick to point out, just six months ago, I was one of those people. I was just as quick to point out to her that it was only five months ago, and I am still their size technically. Then as we continued the conversation, I must have struck a nerve, she reminded me, everyone doesn't have all day to work out and worry about their food consumption. Then here it came, some people have a job you know. There it was staring us right in the hairy eyeball, the J O B topic. Sometimes I wonder which of us had the brain tumor, brain surgery and stroke, her, or I. I have spent the last three years of my life consumed by the effect of this whole brain defect situation. There isn't a waking moment when I don't deal with something related to it. It was the stroke and disability that put me on this journey in the first place. I just seen the social security disability doctor on September 24, 2016 when I got home from Vegas and he confirmed that I am still disabled. So again, what am I supposed to do? Sit in a chair and watch my life pass by? I will save you the hassle, Bull Shit!! I have come too far in a short time to quit now; I have increased my will power muscle by 10-fold. I am on a mission that believe you me, get on board or get the hell out of my way. My life is far from being over and until they lay me to rest, I plan on continuing to fight on. My point to her was not just to the fat people at Logan's, anyone struggling with their weight. It's not too late, No, your results may not be as quick as this 51-year-old stroke survivor, but baby steps then. First things first, chose to start your journey. Second, figure out a plan that works within your lifestyle. Three no matter what happens, stay the course, see it till the end. Feel blessed that you live in the USA, there are hundreds of plans, programs, and products to choose from. I think this is where I struck a nerve last night. So, we are switching internet companies and our service won't be activated until Thursday this week. We have been without Internet at the house for about a week now. In today's world that is an eternity. I have the luxury of taking my laptop to the Tamerac with me and using my cool down time to sit in the comfortable chairs and type away. Not so much for my wife. So, last night after dinner, we took a ride to the local coffee shop and used their internet. I caught up on the book and she researched some items and reconnected with Facebook. Lol but after that we stopped by Wal-Mart for a couple of items. Remember I just got done updating the book, so my mind was still swimming in healthy thoughts. So, as we perused down a couple of the food aisles. I couldn't help to stop and actually look at the labels on some of the items I used to just throw into the cart. I think that is where her nerve problem started to get aggravated. Then we stopped at the glass case where the nerve went into full out pain fest. No, I am not talking about the ice cream glass case, for me it was worse. My youngest daughter used to be vegetarian, so this glass case housed the Morning Star fake meat selection. But just next to this case was a case that stored a new frozen product, I have never seen before. They were Paleo diet frozen meals and individual Paleo frozen food items. I guess I must be getting ready to start or something, because you would have thought they said my baby was ugly or something. I don't know if it was the fact that one of their burritos was $5.00 or that the item I looked at had 340 calories for grains and chicken I believe. Not sure what Paleo diet plan they were following but I didn't think chicken was an option. I'm not 100% sure, I have not done a ton of research on it. I just know for $5.00 you could make a much better and healthier food selection. Again, though, at least we live in a country that gives us the opportunity to spend our money as foolishly as we want, when and if we want. Just saying.

L, LaHooser!!! For someone that has spent their whole life trying to win, I find it very difficult accepting that I'm a loser. I don't mean it in a bad way, but as a weight loser. It is still weird switching over to the dark side really. It wasn't that long ago in the evolution of our fads, where people would hold up a L on their foreheads as the universal loser sign. That sign and the word loser still resonates with me. I'm not sure I will ever fully accept being a loser. Like I said, for my entire life, I wanted to be a winner. I am just a little competitive OK; bull shit I am a big fat competitor. Now add that to my anal compulsive tendencies. And that explains why I am such an ass about winning. Lol In my defense, I have also experienced a lot of personal loss in my life too. So, this to weighs on the willingness to accept the word loser in the weight loss game. I do believe that this for the most part is a game. A serious game for most of us, but a game none the same. We play it daily, on what we eat, how we exercise. Our general lifestyle. It is all interconnected. I wrote this morning on the traumatic experience I had this morning when I found out that I gained two pounds. For some people, that's like no big deal and I know for a person my size, that's a healthy bowel movement, so no big deal. But to a fat guy trying to mend trust issues with his body. It was more of a statement, from my body. Basically, my body was putting me on notice, that it was still calling the shots. It wasn't happy with me, for cutting back its food intake and cutting back its workout regimen. Yes, I did a bigger variety of exercises last week, but my body is not sold on the changes yet. Now without sounding like a lunatic. I almost felt like Syble, this morning. In my anger and denial this morning after the weight gain, I was trying to figure out my next move. My mind was saying, do spinning class again and work harder. My heart was saying don't listen to that guy, he didn't mean it, and my body was saying, go ahead bring it. You thought you walked funny after that last spinning class you put me through, do it again, try me. So, to keep the peace, I stayed the course. I looked at the journals and figured out where I think I went wrong and I will make adjustments and see how we do next week. See weight loss is a game, sometimes you can't win for losing. Just saying

Living my life to live: I wrote about this earlier in the book on the importance of living your life. We I realized this morning as I sat in the hot tub, I was living my life right now so hopefully I could live my life longer and healthier. The more I thought about it and the evolution of who we are. We are born into this crazy world with nothing, as we grow and learn we begin to accumulate things. I was going to say knowledge, but we accumulate a lot more than just knowledge, we pick up habits along the way too. As we move into our 30's and 40's we start to apply the knowledge that we learned into our daily life and begin to open our wings and fly freely. Then our 50's and 60's hit and it's time to start slowing down and take it easier. We start reconnecting with our bodies, whether we want to or not. This is about the time our bodies start breaking down from all the abuse we have put on it over the years. If we are fortunate enough to make it into our 70's and 80's time doesn't play such a factor anymore. Remember when we were young, we lived and died by the clock. Have you ever noticed the older generation does things on their own agenda? Not being a member of that club yet, I had to ask some members why that was. The best answer I got, was "Son when you get to my age, time is all we have left to give." I liked his answer, when you live by the clock, you die by the clock. The key is time management and spending enough time on you. Remember you are that big fleshy thing that holds everything together around you. Just saying. My typical day is up at 4am, gym by 5am, work till 11:30, home by noon, eat my second meal, housework, prepare third meal and eat about 5pm, after meal, go for a walk. In bed by 8pm. Rinse and repeat. Exciting stuff. I plan the excitement in the next journey.

You're not the boss of me!! I don't know if it is my age, or the fact that I have owned most of the business's I have worked for. But I have a big problem with someone barking orders at me. Case in point, I have been taking more exercise classes at the Tamerac the past couple of weeks. Remember up until I lost the first 100 lbs. I did it all on my own. Listening to my body and flying by the seat of my pants basically. Since I have started this challenge, I have lost nine pounds in three weeks, but the two pounds I gained last week was the first time in five months that I have gained any weight I wasn't trying to gain. I did put on the water weight at the beginning of the challenge, that I am still trying to shed completely. There are several instructors at the club, but there are only a couple that I enjoy going too. Kate does the classes in the pool and Tracie does the energizer dance class I do on land. Dance class you may be asking? Yes, it is a combination of Zumba, aerobics, and dance. The dance part reminds me that I am still disabled. It is very challenging for my balance and reminds me that I don't have any rhythm any more lol Not that I had very much of it before the stroke, but at least back then I wasn't terrorized to be on the dance floor. I have seen some of the other instructors in action and I was never in the army and don't plan to start now. I have been in a couple of my regular classes, when you can tell the instructor wasn't feeling it and the class energy dragged. I guess at that point you have three options. One just go with it and chalk it up for just another day completed. Two, get up and make the walk of shame out of the class. (not a good walk by the way) or three depending on the class size and if you know most of the people in the class. Have fun with it, over exaggerate the exercises, no, don't go bat shit crazy, but have more fun than usual, maybe the instructor will feed off your energy and find their groove again. Just a thought, you are already there, get the most out of being there. Just saying

Raindrops keep falling on my head. Another adjustment I have had to make since coming back to Michigan is adjusting to the weather. I was in Vegas for nearly three months and rain altered my work out twice. It seems that it has rained every other day since I have been back here. Needless to say, it has put a damper on my after-dinner walks. Yes, I could go buy a wetsuit, or use an umbrella or make a second trip to the Tamerac for the day. No none of them are as easy as putting my shoes on and walking out my front door, but they are all viable options. Along with those options is going to Wal-Mart and walking there or at the local grocery store I guess. I believe I could go walk at the local school still after school hours. The point is, there are options if I chose. The moral of the story is changing your excuses into options will increase your chances for success immensely. On a side note, this is where building that will power comes into play. Walking through the bakery of your local grocery may be a pretty challenging feat, if you can refrain from making any purchases while making your rounds, will also affect the success of your journey too.

Show me the money!! One of the biggest ways to lose motivation, is lack of follow through. I mentioned that I started a fall challenge at the Tamerac, the place I work out at. It started on October 4th, 2016 basically the same day I started my second journey to the second 100 lb. loss. I joined the challenge being skeptical, remember I have worked pretty independently through the first 100 lbs. But after reading the flyer they had posted around the club, I thought it might not be a good motivational tool to keep me moving. One of the things that caught my eye about the challenge was weekly prizes for the winning team per week. Trust me this is not the "Biggest Loser" we are not looking at big time prizes. I think week one's prize was a $5.00 credit to your account. Like I said, that's not going to bump me up to a higher tax bracket or anything. So here we are starting week three of the contest and they have not updated anything so far. Personally, I lost six lbs. Week one and five lbs. In week two. So, 11 lbs. Total, not too shabby but I am always looking to do more. The moral of the story is it is better to under promise and under produce, then to over promise and under produce. At least if you set an expectation that you can deliver, good bad or indifferent. You keep the faith of your contestants that are sweating their ass's off and doing the challenges you have set forth for them, while they fly in the dark not knowing how they are doing in the challenge they signed up for. Ok, rant over.

Pardon the interruption: Remember the rant when I talked about the community pool? To me community means, come, use, and return things the way you found them, Right? Just one thing I missed and that would be respect the other members working around you. Every other day I do a lower body workout in the pool. Half of the exercises I do for this workout require me to utilize the ladder in the deep end of the pool to stabilize my body. Require may be a strong word for this application, the use of the ladders arms, makes the workout more enjoyable. How's that? Typically, there is a group of ladies that workout about the same time as I do, this is me not judging, but I use the term workout loosely. It never fails I will be deep into my work out when one of the ladies finds it necessary to come over and ask me to move while she tries with all her might to climb the ladder, so she doesn't have to walk as far to put her noodle away. Seriously, are the 30 or so extra steps it would take you to walk to the shallow end of the pool, going to push you into overload? Again, this is not me judging, just stating a fact. Being a good neighbor carries a lot of weight in a community of members with a lot of weight when you learn to play nice early. It's not like I yelled CANNONBALL!! And jackknifed in the middle of their gossip session or anything like that!! Yet!!

Super-size this, value size!! We live in a fat world right now. I know I have said it over and over again that we are fat people living in a skinny person's world. But we as fat people need to be compassionate to the needs of skinny people too. I am sure when they go to the market and see jumbo sized items for slightly over the regular price of their sized items, they probably curse us too. I am sure they are thinking the same thing I am, "no wonder they are fat?" Right. I agree with you skinny mother of two that never gained six ounces. That was bad of me, but it's true the six-ounce comment... no the part about the market. Why would you pay more to get less of the product you want? That's just stupid, right? Wrong!!! Research has proven somewhere I am sure, that we will consume more of a product if we have more of it available. Case in point, how many of us will damn near use vice grips to squeeze the last speck of toothpaste out of a tube of toothpaste whether we have another tube available or not, but if we have that industrial strength sized gallon o toothpaste, we goop it on like it's the fourth meal of the day. Ok don't lie to me, who else was pissed at McDonald's when they changed the box for the 20-piece chicken Mc-nuggets into two 10 piece boxes? I was, not gonna lie, it was something about opening the box and seeing all 20 of those delicious golden treats just waiting to be dipped into that sweet n sour sauce. I'm sorry I regress on occasions. It's true though. Companies have done the math, it doesn't cost that much more for them to increase the size of the container and add a few more fruity pebbles and squeeze a couple of more pennies out of us and they look like the good guys, by putting 25% more. Like we needed the 75% of the crap in the first place. I told you the story of "Possible Pat" he threw all of his food away and walked to the store whenever he was hungry. Out of sight out of mind, if you don't have all this extra food screaming "EAT ME!!!" all the time, wouldn't that be easier. On a side note, if you think about it. Aren't the food manufactures breaking their own rules? If they keep getting us more fat with the jumbo sizes, won't we die faster and not be able to buy more of their products over the remainder of our brief life?

Make the rest of your life the best of your life!! That sounds easy, doesn't it? How is that possible if you keep living in the past? As an old washed up jock, we all live for our glory days, whatever they may have been. I guess if you were the super bowl mvp, or put in the hall of fame or won the Nathan's Hot Dog Eating Competition for us fat guys. I guess those might be worth recalling. For us regular schmoes the best years need to be ahead of us, because there really not many great ones behind us. What is stopping you from making your future your best? Age, weight, health, money? Did I miss anything? EXCUSES is all I heard!! Age, yes your age is going to change, but other than adapting to your environment and figuring out how to do it best, age is just a number. Weight, weight can change also, remember this is a lifestyle change, if you don't like the weight you are at change it! Health, health at least a good portion of it is controlled by your nutritional intake. Control your weight and diet and help control your health. Money, money will always be an issue, there never seems to be enough of it to go around. Two words, financial planner. The sooner in life you get connected with a knowledgeable financial planner the longer your money should last. Before you call B.S. on my financial advice, I was an Assistant Vice President for Flagstar Bank, and banking manager of the year for them in 2005. I did hold my series six license as well for five years. So, I do know a little bit about this subject as well. The moral to this rant, for every excuse we can make that ultimately can hold us back, YOU need to find a solution to make it possible. Remember those 10 two letter words "If It Is to Be It Is Up to Me!" Make the rest of your life the best of your life!!

What age are we? I have said over and over, I am a product of the 60's, I am younger than the "Baby Boomers and younger than the "Depression age" or the Golden Oldies." I think I am too old to be a "Millennial "and thank God I am not a member of the "entitlement generation." Does that make me a member of generation "X" or even a member of the "Pepsi" generation? I guess in the long run it doesn't change who I am or what I am as long as I live my life according to works best for me. Society in general loves to make up cute titles to call people without ever considering what effect it might have on them. It is sad in a way that we just can't be the person that we were born to be without being stereotyped into a category to make some statistical numbers freak happy that everyone is accounted for, like who is counting anyway? You might be wondering where this rant is going? So, get to it fat guy!! Okay, so I was at the gym today sitting in the café area, typing on the book, when a mother and her son sat down at the table next to me. The mother was getting ready to drop her son off at the daycare the gym provides for its members. I couldn't help to notice that the boy was still in his pajamas, which was a little odd since it was 9:30 am but remember I don't judge. Just my luck on of her Millennial friends came over for a chat, so I got some good intel for the book. The mother ordered a double espresso from the café, while she ordered the son a Pop Tart, he was all good with the bug juice he was sipping on, I guess. As he fixated on the IPad he was watching I heard the mom explain to her friend that he was learning Spanish on the IPad.

The program he was watching was designed to teach kids Spanish as they watched the program. Before you scream B.S. I kinda already figured that one out. Supposedly the program doesn't actually teach them this cool trick now that they are under five years of age, she explained to the other mother that, the process just subliminally stores the words they are learning in their sub conscious, until such time as they have Spanish class in school, then the words resonate with the child as if they have known them for years. Isn't that special? Trust me, it took all I could do not to scream out Bull Shit, but I controlled myself, instead I was trying to control my emotions about the child's nutritional habits being formed at that very moment. Kudos to the mom, for making the effort to get to the gym and work on your health, but a double espresso before you work out? That's a bit risky, isn't it? Then we have little Johnny or whatever his name was, learning Spanish at age four, because this is his most impressionable years, says the IPad program thingy, so let's teach him that it is ok to go to the gym in your pajamas, eat a pop tart and drink a bug juice. That covers about 0 of the daily recommended food groups. It almost nips the corner in one of the categories if you squint your eyes and stretch the truth a bit. The younger you teach your kids to eat healthy, the longer your child will eat healthier. That is a proven fact. Think about it, even if they only eat healthy while they live in your house, from 0-18, it would take until year 37 for them to eat unhealthier than when they lived with you and that is if they decided to go bat shit crazy for the 18 years after they moved out. See my point?

Moms waiting for her check? So, I was sitting in the hot tub this morning, pondering the age-old question? How the hell did this happen to us and then it hit me like a slap on the back of my head from my dad at the dinner table. It was the extinction of the stay at home mom. We forget how much work mom's put in when we were kids. Think about it, she cooked, cleaned, did laundry, patched us up, taught us how to cook, how to show love, ride a bike, helped us with homework, was our Dr. Phil, before he was known. A taxi service to us and our friends. cheerleader at all our games, dance instructor, personal assistant and for some of us our first best friend. Last but certainly not least, she did all this for little or no compensation and thanks at all, this was her tradeoff for being a mother and giving up her dreams to be a mother and wife for us. I would have to think by the late 80's is when the big transformation took place to dual income households and the stay at home mom and dads became more scarce. Now it seems to be a rarity if a family is fortunate enough to have a stay at home parent. This is also when the term "Super Mom" was invented, this is a term for a mom, that has her shit so much together that the rest of the ladies on the block despises her. She does all the tasks a regular mom does, but she also works a full-time job too. Pretty insane if you think about it. The late 80's is also when the breakdown of the family unit really started to rear its ugly head. Fast food restaurants, started to boom, full service restaurants, started to expand their carryout services. More people started eating out then ate at home and if they ate at home, most of them were eating take out. As a product of the 60's that lived through all the decades leading to the current decade. I apologize for anything I did to perpetuate any of these practices for the youth of today. Yes, I have been alive for so many great inventions, computers, cell phones, the internet, satellite television, skype, google, Facebook. Lol But, with all the good there still is the bad, MSG, high fructose corn syrup, Aids, $30 billion in debt. Pollution, global warming, and the list goes on. Through all this one thing remains constant. Food! Mothers start us off on our first meals, whether you were breastfeeding or not. Mom was our primary food giver FOREVER!!! When we lost her as this important link in the food chain of life, that is really when the fat hit the fan. Just saying. I know my mom got a big fat retroactive check when she hit those pearly gates. I think God had to take out a loan to cover that check after what me and my siblings put her through in our lifetime.

You know you can be to overprotective, right? TWO Remember the part where I am not Dr. Phil, nor am I Dr. Seuss. I am just a fat guy, with years of experience being fat and a ton of nieces and nephews and great nieces and nephews. My oldest nephew is 46, and my youngest niece is eight. So, I run the gamut on experience there too. This rant will be brief, because every parent has their own parenting philosophy and the fact that when you try to interject your own personal philosophies when they are not asked for, panties get in a bunch. So, most of the time I just sit back and watch the action. You know the do as I say not as I do theory of parenting, doesn't really work, right? Maybe it does when they are in front of you, but get them alone, with their cousins and if these walls could talk, begins. Where do you think the phrase "chip off the old block" and "the apple doesn't fall that far from the tree." Or even "Why doesn't your family tree branch?" I apologize for that one, remember I live in the sticks and I digress. Getting back to your kids, they don't miss anything, you may think they don't know your little secrets, but trust me, they are just working on the angles to see when they can use them against you for their biggest bang for the buck. Case in point, one Sunday dinner, my in-laws we up from down state, we were just wrapping things up and my oldest daughter, being about nine at the time, pipes up with I know what the "F" word means. Being shocked that she even brought that up in the first place and in the company of my in-laws was horrific for myself and my wife. So, we did what every other good Christian parent would do and said, Andrea, I think you must be mistaken. Unfortunately for me she said no, mother. "daddy says it all the time when he is mad." Needless to say, neither her or I had any dessert that evening. Kids say the darndest things. Lol I have another niece that has been sheltered from soda, and sweets pretty much her entire life. That is a great thing in theory, but wait until she starts getting her freedom and venturing out with her friends. This is where the fat hits the fan. How quick will it be before she discovers the many flavors of unhealthy food choices awaiting her. Sure, the words sugar overload come to mind, but in my mind so does the resentment from her on her parents from keeping these secrets from her for so long. That's why I am so pro in moderation. Give your kids the real thing but offer them the healthy choice as well and guide them from there. If we try to control them while they are under our control, there is a better chance of them being out of control when they are on their own. Love them for all that they are and guide them to all they can be…

Be careful what you wish for!! I really never talked about my surgery that much. I guess it really doesn't matter how I got here, it really just matters what I do to get better and move on. To say I was not pleased with the way everything ended after my surgery and stroke would be a monumental understatement of biblical proportion. No, it wasn't the end of the world, but it was the end of my life as I knew it. Not to dwell, moving on. So, one of the fun yearly events, I get to partake in every year since the surgery is a lovely brain MRI. No, it's not painful but two things that really suck about them. One the table and machine are not designed to accommodate fat people like I was, so up until the one I did this September. I was stuffed into the machine like a sardine in a can. This year not so much, it was comfortable for a change. Second, if you have never had the pleasure of having a head MRI, you don't know what you are missing. I generally have a headache for the following three to four days. I don't know if it's the jackhammer sound pulsating through my head or the magnetic waves messing with the plate in my head. Either way again, it sucks. Like I said, I have these yearly now, at least I have for the past three years. Generally, I have them in August, but since I was out of the state, I had it in September. I had the test, a couple days later I got an email from my health website that my results were in and ready for my viewing. I went to the site, logged in and proceeded to read the report. Everything seemed to check out with no changes. So, I was good with that, in the meantime the doctor's office called and said that the surgeon that did my brain surgery reviewed my report and wanted to talk to me. With the history, I have with him, I wasn't too quick to call back. So today I get a call from his nurse and she leaves me a voicemail dr. wants me to have another MRI. WTF. So of course, being the calm level headed, rational fat assed product of the sixties. My mind springs into action and start texting my wife. My wife is in the medical field and she also works in the radiology department that I had my MRI done at. You would think she would have heard something if it wasn't good, Right? Then I started thinking, what if the tumor is back causing something supernatural allowing to work out as hard as I want for as long as I want and never get tired or sore. Kinda like John Travolta in Phenomenon. Ya, we can all dream, Right? Oh, wait he dies at the end of the movie, I think I will pass on that ending and I lived happily ever after, brain tumor free. Now I feel better. So, I got that call about 10am but didn't see I missed the call till 11:30am. The message said she wouldn't be back in the office until 1pm. So, you can imagine the crap that was going through my head for that long grueling 90 minutes or 54,000 seconds. Whichever seems longer. So 1:20 comes, I needed to be fashionably late calling right, I do have a rep. somewhere. So, I call into the number she left me and I brace for the worst. The nurse answers the phone and say, dr. reviewed the MRI reports and everything looks good, you don't have to have another scan for two years. Seriously, how did things go from dr. wants you to have another scan done to see you in two years in a matter of a couple of hours? Here I was hoping to get answers on why I can still do what I am doing daily and the call was to tell me I didn't need to be scanned again for two years. I guess I should be relieved that the news was positive, but now I have a headache. LOL

Never stop learning: Every generation has things to offer, just because we don't do things the same way as they did exactly before us. It's called evolution. For example, I was walking behind an older gentleman at the gym today and he was using a manual clicker in his right hand to count his step. The clicker looked familiar being an old baseball coach and all. It looked like the one I used to use to keep track of my pitcher's pitch count. So, being the smart assed inquisitive person I am I said coach what's with the clicker? First of all, "he said no one had called him coach in a long time," but then yes, he admitted to be an old baseball coach from years gone by. I asked so what's his story with it, he said "his doctor wanted him to walk three miles a day or the equivalent of three miles in steps a day." So, I was in the talkative mood today and being the "rain man" that I am with numbers, I said so how do you track your 12,672 steps you need? And Wapner at 3pm definitely 3. Without skipping a beat, he must have been a smart ass in his day too. He said every 10 feet I hit the clicker. I start with all zero's and hit the strike button first every time I get to 10 step. When the strikes fill up I click the next button. When I fill up the strikes, balls, out and 12 innings, I have 12,0000 steps then I only need 624 more steps to hit my goal. I said that was cool, but you know I had to mess with him, I said you know they make things that count all these things automatically for you, right? And he said yep and I said and? He said, "this was a gift from the first team I ever coached and I told them I would use it forever." Son forever isn't over yet for me and by the way it keeps my mind working, is that such a bad thing". I said it never is and I thanked him for his time and his lesson for the day. Just because there are things out there that can make a job easier, doesn't always mean it makes the job any easier in the long run. Just saying.

So, where does the fat go? I told you over and over again, I don't have a degree in anything related to what I am doing here, remember. I just get up daily and go do. So, I was wondering where does the fat go? I'm not trying to be a smart ass here either. This is just me being my skeptical cynical self and asking everyone to think about this one. I get the fact that fat is made up of calories, this magical little chemical that we can't actually see, but it's in everything but water basically. On a side note I call bull shit of the water weight, while we are on the subject. I learned that my body carries on average four pounds of water weight on a daily basis. I generally weigh myself at the end of the day, basically to test this theory. Every night I weigh four pounds lighter than I do the following morning when I weigh in. It kinda pisses me off, actually it really pisses me off, just saying, okay back to the rant. So pretty much all food has these invisible calories that make up fat. So, we eat the food and gain weight and that weight converts to fat. Okay I get that, so then we exercise and burn calories and in turn we burn fat. Okay check. So, we burn fat and lose weight, so where does it go? Does it turn to water and we sweat it out? Does it turn to waste and we poop it out? I know I haven't thrown up lately, so I know I'm not losing it there either. The reason I say this, is that I have lost a quarter of my body weight in a little over 100 days, I would think I would have extra hanging skin on me. But that is not the case, anywhere on me. So, where did it go? Everyone other than my pool Goddess Kate, downplays the benefits of the pool to me. They still find it too hard to fathom that I have transformed my body so quickly walking in the pool. Is there an explanation anywhere out there from anyone that may have the answer for me? Please email me this information to fatcamper1@gmail.com and thank you for your time.

Where did they go? I find it pretty amazing, the people I have met along the journey. I never really considered myself to be introverted or shy by any means, but ever since the stroke, I guess I have been more reluctant to strike up a conversation with people I don't really know why, self-conscious about my brain to mouth disconnect I get sometimes I guess. Case in point, I was 50 years old, when I started my journey back in June at the Resort Villas in Nevada. I didn't know anyone but my sister and brother in-law at that time. As I continued my daily workout routine at the pool and on my walk to the pool. I met all kinds of wonderful people, with a lot of common interests as I did, but the biggest thing we had in common was everyone had someone that was fat. Not a chunky friend or family member, but a fat one. At first, they were all P.C. about it, until I referred to myself as being fat, then that kinda broke the fat barrier and the floodgates of lard flowed freely. I was fine with it, I told you I am so done with sugar coating it and tip toeing around the problem. It's time we started addressing the big elephant in the room. Everyone wants equal rights these days, then they better be able to handle the truth. The saddest part to everyone's story, was most of the time the fat person died. It didn't matter how old they were, what economic or religious background they were from. Black, white, Hispanic. Obesity does not discriminate. It will kill you and move on to your relatives next. Think about it, grieving people eat food to comfort their loss, it is tradition to bring food to the family that loses someone. That's ok, it is a tradition we have done for centuries, why stop now. I know, I hear you kill the fat guy, that insensitive prick, trying to take our wake food away. I am not trying to take anything away. I am just stating a fact. Our lives revolve around food and we wonder why people are disappearing from our lives, Healthy eating habits, help prolong life, why do we wait until we are near death or lose someone dear to us before we chose to get healthy? Just saying.

Failure is not an option!! No, this is not a scare tactic, this is not a treat. This is not directed at the skinny people I haven't totally offended yet, that might still be reading this book. This is for the ones of us that have had a major defect, such as a stroke, heart attack, diabetes, high blood pressure. You know the healthy fat people. NOT. This is not the doctor speaking, this is the same fat guy that you have been ignoring for the entire book so far, so why should you start now? Every day you wait or waste, is one less day you have to make the rest of your life the best of your life. Seriously, we live in one of the weirdest times ever for me. Obesity is at an all-time high, but if you watch television late at night or on weekends, there are plenty of infomercials about starving kids all over the world. It is so unfortunate that we can't take the fat that we lose and give it to the kids that need it the most. But wait there is!! In my Don Pardo voice. If you are so set in your ways to keep buying food, why not take the food you have to buy and donate it to the local food pantry? Or if you are still eating fast food, because you said screw this fat guy, he is not the boss of me, I am a grown ass man. If I want a double heart attack and a side stroke, with a jumbo diet soda to wash it down. I am going to have it damnit. Hey go for it big guy, did you ever wonder why fast food restaurants accept credit cards but never offer you one of their credit cards? Because they know your life expectancy isn't that long. They will sell you a gift card, because they don't care if you use that after you pay them for it. Okay back to the rant. If you are so hell bent on going to the fast food places, why not buy gift cards, and give them to the people in need. You know the people on the corner that are asking for donations? Give them the gift cards, they have no cash value and they have to use them for food and without saying "I use that food term loosely" I do. That leads me into my next rant. When you find, yourself positioning your stuffed animals around your pity party table. Just remember as bad as you think you may have it. There is someone out there, that has it worse than you. I wasn't going to go here, because I am not proud of this, but it is a part of how I got here. So, in order to come clean and admit my mistakes, here goes. I have gone bankrupt twice, I have lost three businesses, two houses, five cars, one time-share, my wife and one daughter. I could give two shits about the first 10 items on the list, but the last two broke my heart and losing my training business took my passion and ability to coach. The stroke almost took my will to live but this journey is slowly restoring that for me. I think back and on my darkest days and there was still someone out there that had it worse than me. I thank God, every day for the things I have in my life, but I also thank him for everything that are not things also. Amen!!

Challenges can be to challenging. Week one is in the books for the Tamerac "Fall into fitness challenge" I learned a lot more about myself this week. I tried to conform to the workout regimen that was required by the challenge to earn the most points for your team. I learned that my body doesn't like it very much when I stop listening to it also. According to their scale I lost six lbs. This past week. According to the way my body is reacting, I lost way more in trust with my body then weight that was recorded. If you haven't noticed this about me yet, I kinda jump into things with three feet. I really don't have a half speed. The way I look at it, "life is too short to waste time" plus "I will rest when I am dead." pretty much my go to mottos. So, I hit it pretty hard last week. I doubled up and even tripled up some of my class workouts. I did an hour spinning class and I haven't been able to sit right since. I spent well more time in the sauna than I ever have and pretty much was hungry all week. I know my body has to be saying, "what the hell are you trying to do to me fat guy?" "We just let you lose 100 lbs. Without ever getting sore, why are you killing us now?" I don't have an answer for it. Why do we do that? Never satisfied with a good thing, always needing more, for what? For me I guess I keep hearing everyone telling me the second hundred isn't going to come off as easy as the first 100. So, I feel the need to push it harder. I should have continued the same regiment and seen if there was any drop off before I made such a drastic change. I am going to spend the rest of the week repairing the trust issues with my body and start listening more. I think that might help restore the harmony again. I will keep you posted.

Well, the challenge is over and I would have to say it was a monumental failure for me. I think I have set myself back months. My body is not happy with me, my mind is not happy with me and I am not happy either. I spent the last six weeks or so working in someone else's world. My mind never bought into the concept of working towards the point system set up by pretty much skinny people. The instructors that put this program together are fit people that lumped everyone together. You know when you weigh more individually, then each of the top three teams in the challenge, you are pretty much screwed. The top three teams in the challenge are all fitness fanatics. I guess I should have did a little more research before entering the contest. Every week I weighed in I was disappointed, they didn't understand why. On four of the six weeks I lost weight, but the most I lost in any week was five pounds. Some people might think that was great, but I know where I have been, and I know how hard I worked every week and what I put into my body, to not see results I am satisfied with is disappointing. I originally set a goal to lose 50 lbs. for the challenge and to gain five pounds is devastating. Life goes on though, I will continue to watch what I put in my mouth and begin a new workout regimen when I get to Va. Beach. I leave for Virginia Beach on Monday to spend a couple month's with my daughter Andrea and hopefully get her started on a healthier lifestyle.

Tip Last: Dear fat person, sorry that you wasted your money on this book. There is no magic potion to cure your fatness, this book is about my journey on how I lost it, you're not ready to start your journey if you don't want to take the time to read how I did it and take some friendly advice. Take Care Love Big Sexy